FORMULA 14

Jordan Church
Formula 14

Published by Spines
ISBN 979-8-89569-873-0

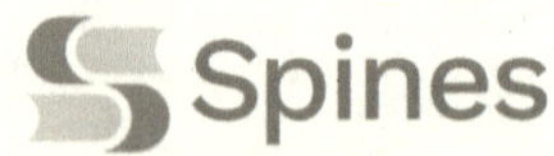

FORMULA 14

THE LAST WEIGHT LOSS BOOK YOU WILL EVER NEED

JORDAN CHURCH

CONTENTS

SECTION FOUR
THE PATH AHEAD

DISCLAIMER

The information on the following pages has not been evaluated by the Food and Drug Administration and is not meant to replace the services of health professionals or to be a substitute for medical advice from your Doctor. You are advised to discuss health challenges and questions with your health care professional for weight loss and improved health, especially matters that may require a diagnosis or medical attention.

This book is dedicated to my wife Marie, and my babies: Lily, Kate, and Finn. I love you. Also, all of the original Formula 14 Ambassadors, and the people who helped me as I developed the Formula 14 system: Helen Schroder, Nick and Sharon Church, Lane Penry, Jay Church, Lawton Jordan, Robert Abercrombie, Max Holland, Marco Sanchez, Robert Hicks, Jason Brady, and David Carter.

I would also like to dedicate this book to anyone who has struggled with their weight. Congratulations! You are about to learn the Formula 14 system and the powerful strategies you can use to eliminate excess poundage! I want to offer a glimmer of hope to those of you who, like me, have been tormented by obesity and weight challenges for most of their lives. You can make the changes necessary and erase the negative impact it has had on your life. There is a way out, and I am honored that you are taking the time to let me share my experiences with you. I hope that we can meet some day and you can share your success story with me and/or carry the message to others as a Formula 14 Ambassador!

THANK YOU!

Thank you for buying my book! If you want access to additional tools and videos, please go to formula14community.com to get updates and stay in touch.

BATTLES OF THE BULGE

You've got to get yourself together
You got stuck in a moment
And you can't get out of it
Don't say that later will be better
Now you're stuck in a moment
And you can't get out of it…

Stuck in a Moment---------U2

I am not a doctor. I am not a dietitian. I am not a psychologist. You may consider this bad news and decide to put the book down. It's not for you. On the flip side, me not being a psychologist, doctor, or dietitian could also work in your favor. If you have struggled with being overweight, who do you think can help you more? The person who was 361 pounds and morbidly obese but is now at a healthy weight and maintaining it, or the man or woman who was a track star in high school, has never been even a pound overweight—in fact, they've been slightly underweight their entire life—went to college for 12 years, got a master's in exercise physiology and nutrition, and has now written a book that tells you to eat more salads and grilled chicken, take up yoga three times a week, and lift weights twice a week? A person that has never dealt with emotional eating or woken up in the morning obsessing about what they are eating for lunch and dinner that day?

So, this introduction delves deeply into my past and my decades-long struggle with obesity and weight loss. I thought it necessary to explain that I am not a doctor or a dietitian, just an average person who has had a decades-long battle with obesity. In some ways, my story may mimic yours, and hopefully, you will also find answers with Formula 14.

Regardless, if you are the type of person who started reading this and said to yourself, "What is this guy carrying on about? Give me the strategies I need and stop rambling on!" then you may want to skip to the first chapter.

I have struggled with weight problems my entire life. I have always loved to eat, and some of the best times my family had were around the dinner table. My grandmothers made delicious meals with dishes that would keep you coming back for more and more. After a two-week visit to my grandparents' house, my mom and dad were always mortified when they picked up my brother and me. "You look like all you've done for the past two weeks is stuff your face," Mom would say. Indeed, each summer day was a sprint from one meal to the next, and when we all gathered for the holidays, wow! Thanksgiving Day was a marathon eating session that left the entire family happily stuffed—so much so that naps were in order. Then we would wake up and have pound cake, chocolate delight, or pumpkin pie smothered in whipped cream.

As a child, I was fascinated with bodybuilders and miracle

exercise programs advertised in the back of comic books. I was pudgy and not very athletic, so I was enamored with the pictures of Arnold Schwarzenegger and other early bodybuilding superstars. I owned a book about Charles Atlas and even ordered a free-hand exercise system when I was around ten years old. I lost the small booklet on a family vacation and was devastated. I had finally discovered the secret that was going to make me as strong as a tiger, and now it was lost forever!

I went to Europe with my uncle and cousin when I was twelve years old and was already talking about dieting. The delicious meals in Germany and Switzerland were too tempting for any real change, but I remember talking about dieting the whole time. I talked so much that my uncle finally said, "You need to make a decision about whether or not you are going to diet."

I remember going to Weight Watchers™ with my mother. A friend of mine was there, accompanying his mother to her weigh-in. I was embarrassed and humiliated. My parents also put me on Slim Fast™ and the Hilton Head Metabolism Diet™. I succeeded and failed at both extremely well. I would lose weight, but once I returned to my old eating habits, the weight came back rapidly, plus a few extra pounds.

My weight fluctuated up and down for years until I fell in love with running as a teenager. I was never a fast runner, but I could keep a steady pace and loved the sense of accomplishment I would feel after a long run. By the time I was twenty, I was in the best shape of my life and even ran a few half-marathons. I became a vegetarian for over five years, but once I stopped running, my weight began to creep upward.

I was not a healthy vegetarian. I was a vegetarian glutton and ate little or no protein. I thought avoiding meat was better for me, so instead of having bacon and eggs, I would be "healthy" and have a waffle and hash browns. To top it off, I would have two or three Cokes™ or sweet teas during the meal. So, my weight went from an adult low of 157 lbs up into the 180s and then steadily crept up to 361 lbs over the next decade.

Because I had experienced being fit and feeling healthy, and was constantly researching diet and exercise systems, I thought that getting back to a healthy weight would not be much of a problem. "Oh my gosh, I'm 200 pounds! Well, that's no big deal. I know what to do to get healthy... but not today. I want to have a delicious meal... maybe I'll diet tomorrow." Six months later: "Gosh, I'm 218 pounds. No big deal, I know what to do to get lean. But not today, I will research and plan..."

It was during this period that Journal Madness began. I would go to the bookstore, buy an $8.00 journal, document my "last supper" and then write about how the time had finally come to take action. This magical moment of motivation would last until about noon the following day, when fruit gave way to a Big Mac™. I thought that the book *Fit For Life* was a masterpiece, but I never fully realized that pounding fruit from the time I woke up until noon gave me serious carbohydrate cravings.

Then, one Thanksgiving, my dad was losing weight with the Atkins Diet™ and was convinced that it was the answer. His conviction overpowered my belief that excess meat was unhealthy, and I spun off in a new direction in pursuit of a thinner body. Low carb was very effective... for a few weeks. Then, when I started adding back the carbs, it was never the healthier foods recommended, like blueberries, cauliflower, and grapefruit; it was cake, soda, pizza, and fast food. So low carb (or at least my twisted version of it) was not the answer.

I tried every diet: no carb, low carb, fasting, cleansing herbs, workout-centered, and on and on. I was an expert in the current weight loss fad of the day. I could give anyone the strategies to lose weight, but I did not have the willpower or the compelling motivation to consistently use that information on myself.

One Christmas, my sister-in-law, and her husband came from London to visit us at our home in Atlanta. We headed south so that they could experience Walt Disney World and Universal Studios. What should have been a wonderful trip ended up being a nightmare. We shared a hotel room, and my snoring kept everyone awake. When I pass the 280-pound mark, my snoring is like a jackhammer. Each morning was terribly embarrassing as everyone slowly woke up and stared at me through glazed eyes. I could tell what they were thinking: "You kept me awake all night. You are the reason I'll barely be able to keep my eyes open today."

While the snoring was embarrassing, it did not even hold a candle to the Dueling Dragons. The Dueling Dragons were a pair of roller coasters at Universal's Islands of Adventure before the section was converted to a Harry Potter theme. They spiral and twist around each other, giving you the illusion that you are about to collide with the opposing coaster (dragon). One was called Fire, and the other was called Ice. We decided that we would all wait in line to ride the front seats because we would be flying through the air with nothing in front of us, our feet dangling, spinning, and twirling for a thrill ride. When we finally reached the front, we sat down, but when the attendant, a tiny teenage girl, tried to press the padded restraint bar down over me, it wouldn't close. She pressed several times, and then said, "I'm sorry, but you are going to have to move." So she walked me back to the fat seat in front of dozens of people. People who had just witnessed her struggle to shut the seat down over my bombastic belly. We arrived at the fat seat, and there was a petite girl sitting in it. The attendant asked her to move so I could sit there. "But I want to be next to my boyfriend," she said.

So, I would have to wait for the next dragon to ride. The attendant walked me back to a holding area, and everyone standing in line watched me walk in front of them. They had seen the entire episode. It was a walk of shame. But it gets worse. When the next train pulled in, the worker came and got me first, before the gates opened to allow the next group of passengers to sit down. I walked back along the front of the crowd and was placed in the fat seat while everybody watched. With the looks I got, the attendant could have yelled, "Dead man walking," and the crowd would have roared with laughter. She sat me down and pressed the seat over me. The few seconds it took to release the other riders seemed like an hour. I was totally embarrassed... but not embarrassed enough to change my behaviors.

By the time I reached my late thirties, I was still over 300 lbs. and morbidly obese. Overeating, horrible food choices, and lack of exercise almost cost me everything—it was a struggle to get up in the morning. I would drag myself out of bed, quickly make my two-year-old a bowl of cereal, and then fall onto the couch and sleep until she was finished eating. I would doze off in the middle of conversations with friends and family members and had little or no energy by mid-afternoon.

I was so heavy that I had to plant both feet on the ground to push myself out of the car. Imagine being short of breath when you bend over to tie your shoes! I avoided friends and family because I was ashamed of my physical appearance. My obsession with food was destroying my life. Even more terrifying was the certainty that serious health problems were on the horizon. The birth of my second daughter brought my ticking time bomb to the forefront and highlighted my ill-health. I wanted to be a happy, healthy, and energetic dad. My wife was at her wits' end, frustrated with my inability to take care of myself. She had listened to me talk about how I was going to get in shape for years while my stomach swelled to Buddha-like proportions.

Then, a friend told me about a contest she heard her trainer discussing with a manager of her fitness club. She knew I was frustrated and needed to make a change, so she offered to sponsor me in the contest. I entered the Biggest Loser contest through Just Fitness™ and lost 87 pounds in 16 weeks!

How did I do it? I worked out with a personal trainer, saturated my body with water, and followed a moderate nutrition and supplementation guideline. But old habits die hard, and soon after my contest ended, water was replaced with sweet tea and Mocha Frappuccinos, and the weight started to come back. I would realize I was gaining, start walking and eating better, and the weight would fall off again. I stayed in this vicious cycle for almost five years.

Then, one of my upward spirals brought me back to my heaviest weight of 361 pounds! My wife was pregnant, and with all the talk of a new baby in Mommy's tummy, my youngest daughter asked me if I had a baby in my tummy! A family member was seriously ill, and I asked him what I could do to help. He said, "Just take care of your own health." He did not need to elaborate. I started on another meltdown and did okay for a few weeks. Then a foot injury knocked me backward (excuses), my weight loss slowed again, and I began to creep back up towards 300 lbs. I could not go down that path again! My joints were hurting, and I was sure serious health challenges were on the horizon. But it wasn't enough to change!

I had extensive blood work done to test for food allergies and inflammation. I had to face the fact that a real shift in my path required addressing the emotional patterns and attaching new meaning to a healthier journey. My commitment was solidified a week later when my wife told me that our 7-year-old daughter told the neighbors we were carpooling with that my stomach was "yucky and embarrassing." This was devastating but bolstered my resolve, and another meltdown began.

I lost almost 100 lbs in about seven months. I was on a roll! Then, I traveled to Australia to visit relatives, where water was soon replaced with iced coffee with a packet of sugar. Then, iced coffee with nine pumps of classic syrup and a few packets of sugar. At night, I started having Southern Comfort™ Colas, which is a mixed drink in a can. In the mornings, I had hot cross buns. During the day, KFC fries. When I returned from Australia, I had gained over twenty pounds of fat and bloat. What was worse was that the foods I ate before going to Australia, which allowed me to maintain or lose weight every week, would now put a pound or two on my frame every week. The iced coffees returned. Then, two iced lattes every day. Then the convenience(more excuses) of fast food. The months rolled by, and my weight surged upward.

Eight more years of dieting and excuses, hovering between 260 and 361 pounds, usually keeping it under the 300 lb mark but still in the morbidly obese range. Then, reaching the age of 50 in the midst of COVID, and the disease was wreaking havoc on the obese. I knew I needed more life insurance, but I was told I would have to be tested first. I was declined due to high blood sugar and high blood pressure. This started another round of diets and taking my health more seriously, but the same cycle repeated. IF I could just find a way...

Another embarrassing event came when my brother-in-law Shane visited from Australia. We went kayaking down a river on Memorial Day, and I was so heavy the kayak scraped the rocks and flung me out. My wife was mortified as the kayak and paddle drifted towards her. She said she wanted to paddle away and pretend she didn't know me. She was kind, though, and waited with Shane to get me situated again. Five minutes later, another spill. I was too fat to kayak and had to wait on the side of the river for three hours to be picked up. Another humiliating and embarrassing event. But not enough to change.

As a professional matchmaker for twenty years, many of my clients have what we call a "Dating Disruptor." One is “The Dance With Destiny.” This simply means that they have a distorted perception of what relationships are like. Many people think life is like a romantic film where at the end, the two people find each other, and all of the hard work is done, and they skip off into the sunset and live happily ever after. In reality, we know that relationships take dedication and continual effort to make them successful. Another dating disruptor is having unrealistic expectations of your partner (she wants one man made of Hercules and Cyrano - Spin Doctors - Little Miss Can’t Be Wrong). We call this "Interview and Investigate," and then lastly, "Pause and Ponder," where the single person has unrealistic expectations of themselves. "I will date once I am making more money, after I get my degree, and the biggest one: ONCE I LOSE WEIGHT." This was a common theme with my clients, so I made it my mission to find a solution that would work for them.

After decades of struggle, where the bulk of my life was

consumed by fluctuating between 260 and 361 pounds, trapped in morbid obesity and perpetual misery, I started aligning the answers. Throughout most of this time, I hovered around 280 pounds, a staggering 100+ pounds over where I needed to be. Despite experimenting with various strategies, meticulously documenting them, and finding success momentarily, I always faltered in maintaining them. That's when I resolved to craft a comprehensive system that would seamlessly integrate these strategies, guiding me to my ideal weight and ensuring I stayed there for life. The result is a robust system that I firmly believe can empower anyone to achieve similar transformations. You're currently holding that very system in your hands: Formula 14.

Through my research and struggles to find the answers, I found the ANSWERS—the strategy that unlocks the physical and mental methods to end obesity forever: Formula 14!

I was coaching a group of men who all happened to have the ideal weight of 190 lbs. This was my target too, so I joined the friendly competition and applied the 14 Phases of Formula 14! What better person to test this system on than myself? I finally found the path to reach my weight goal. After discovering the simple (not always easy) keys to being lean forever, I had to embrace the journey and realize that emotional and psychological issues would always keep me fat. With the 14 Phases of Formula 14, I am on a different path, and I feel so much better. I am rarely tired, I have the energy to play with my son, and I have high levels of energy throughout the day. I am so much more optimistic about my future and feel that every day is a gift with my improving newfound health.

The three-decade cycle of bouncing between 260 lbs and 361 lbs is over because I implemented all of the components of Formula 14 into my life. Down almost 200 lbs from my heaviest, I am working on adding muscle mass and settling at a healthy and comfortable weight for the rest of my life!

So, let's dive in and discuss the 14 powerful phases of Formula 14. The first four phases alone(the core four) can end obesity in your life FOREVER! Let's get Formula 14 making you lean!

SECTION ONE

THE CORE FOUR

A QUICK NOTE:

Each Chapter will begin with Hour 1/Day 1/Week 1, then Hour 2/Day 2/ Week/2, etc. This simply means if you are implementing the 14 phases of the Formula 14 System quickly over a matter of hours, this is your first hour. If you are implementing it over 14 days, then it's day one. If you are implementing one phase per week, then it's week one. Do not feel confined by this and let it confuse you. The best pace is the one that you stick with, builds momentum, and conquers your weight loss challenges forever!

CHAPTER 1
FORMULA 14 PHASE 1
(HOUR 1/DAY 1/WEEK 1)

YOUR F14

You ain't gone far enough to say
At least I've tried
You ain't worked hard enough to say
Well I've done mine
You ain't run far enough to say
My legs have failed
You ain't gone far enough
You ain't worked hard enough
You ain't run far enough to say
Ain't gonna get any better

Hey Mama - Nathaniel Rateliff

FORMULA 14 CALORIES PER POUND: YOUR F14#

Before we end overeating forever with Formula 14, let me say that I am well aware of the arguments against calorie counting. Calorie counting can overlook the hormonal responses that different foods create in the body. In other words, 200 calories of veggies and olive oil is not the same as 200 calories of M&M's.

Think of a calorie in this context. In a lab, calories are all the same, but in your body, the M&M's will impact your metabolism differently. I have a weakness for sweet tea. It is delicious, delightful, and destructive to the human body. On several occasions, I was losing weight by skipping the sugary tea and just drinking water, but then I slowly started increasing my sweet tea consumption and reducing my intake of water. My weight loss would slow, then plateau, and then creep upward, depending on how much sweet tea I consumed and how little water I was drinking. There were nowhere near enough calories in sweet tea to create that dynamic, but the impact it had on my pH and hormones brought my weight loss to a screeching halt, and I moved from losing pounds to gaining.

Some people have a metabolism that can handle more refined sugar. Mark Haub, a human nutrition professor at Kansas State University, lost 27 pounds in two months while eating Twinkies, Doritos, Frosted Flakes, and other snack cakes. He took a multivitamin and had a protein shake every day, but Haub did not change his exercise level. Haub's metabolism was obviously well-suited for that kind of diet. His bad cholesterol dropped, and his good cholesterol increased, but I would still be concerned about the possible long-term damage from the hydrogenated fat and other chemicals and how this would impact his health.[1]

So, focusing on calories alone is not ideal for everyone – especially those with syndrome X (insulin resistance), which leads to diabetes and a host of other medical conditions. (Excess weight around the midsection can be a sign of pre-diabetes/syndrome X.) That being said, calorie counting can be an effective method to control overeating, which is critical to beating obesity. Overeating has a devastating effect on the entire body. Common sense alone calls into question the habit of constantly stuffing our faces with food. Was the human body made to handle this? What about the salt, the sugar, the meat, the processed foods?

Getting control of the quantity of food you are consuming is critical to losing weight and being healthy. Soon, Formula 14 will become second nature, and you won't need to spend much time counting calories because you'll know them based on the foods you love and your normal eating patterns.

Through calorie counting, Formula 14 ends one of the main drivers of obesity: overeating. So, let's dive into Formula 14 and transform your body FOREVER.

What is your ideal weight? You have to decide on this number before you implement Formula 14. Most people have a number in mind that represents their ideal weight goal. If you have been obese for many years, your bones may have grown thicker to handle the excess weight, and the leanest weight you were as a young adult may not be achievable. If you really don't

---

1. Park. Madison, Twinkie Diet Helps Nutrition Professor Lose 27 Pounds, www.CNN.COM/2010/Health/11/08

have any idea of what your ideal weight goal should be, go to the internet and search "ideal weight chart" and find a number you are comfortable with.

This number may change once you get closer to your goal. Once you have determined what your ideal weight is, you will multiply that number by 14. The resulting number is the maximum number of calories you will have per day for the rest of your life. There are several factors that may shift this number, but here is the formula again:

14 X ideal weight = maximum number of daily calories. This is your F14# and an overarching principle you can use to be lean for the rest of your life. Again, it is:

14 X IDW = MDC (F14#)

There are several reasons this works. First and foremost, if you are 100 pounds overweight, there is no way that 14 calories X your ideal weight will sustain a body that large. So, let's use a 400lb person as an example. They set their ideal weight goal as 200 lbs. 200 X 14 = 2800. 2800 calories cannot sustain a 400 lbs frame. But there is another reason Formula 14 works. With 2800 calories per day, the person in the example can eat ANYTHING they want. They just can't eat EVERYTHING they want. So if they want a Big Mac, large fries, and a large coke, they can have that. In fact, they have only consumed 44% of their daily calories. So if they decide to have a cheeseburger, medium fries, and medium Sprite for dinner, they would only be at 78% of their daily calories and still have room for a peppermint patty or two and some iced coffee.

Now, I can hear the shrieks and cries about how unhealthy

this would be. Remember, we are first addressing over-consumption and making ourselves thinner. We will cover being healthy with the proper hydration, nutrients, supplementation, exercise, and mindset in the later phases of Formula 14.

But if you are following Formula 14, you can try any fad diet and any system of eating, and you will continue to lose weight as long as, when you fall off the fad diet, you fall back into Formula 14 Calories Per Pound and your F14#.

Being able to eat anything you want, just not everything they want, can also help you in the psychological warfare front of the battle of the bulge. If you know that you can have that cake and ice cream after dinner because you ate light during the day, then you have something to look forward to and don't have to feel deprived or guilty. A low-carbohydrate advocate would argue that you are playing with fire to still be dabbling in the tempting world of refined sugar, like a person with drinking problems allowing themselves one shot of whiskey after dinner. One shot becomes two, two becomes four, and all self-control flies out the door! Other issues, such as sugar addiction and blood sugar crashes, can be impacted by the food you eat. We will discuss ideal nutrition in a later phase, for now, just be aware of the challenges that can arise with refined sugar and other carbohydrates.

PLATEAUS AND OBSTACLES ON YOUR JOURNEY

While you are using Formula 14, if you go two consecutive weeks without losing weight, your metabolism may be slowing down. In this case, you may need to multiply your ideal weight by 17 and make that your daily caloric intake one day per week. Seventeen calories per pound is slightly overeating and could kick your metabolism back up.

Another way to address a plateau is to reduce the calories within your F14# and eat within a specific time window, which we will address shortly.

Also, be aware of exercise and the impact it will have on your daily calories. If you are using Formula 14 but start training for a half marathon, you must take into account the daily calories you are burning and adjust accordingly.

One final shift may be required as you get close to your ideal weight. You may have a target of 150 pounds, but once you get to 162, you realize you are at 10% body fat and don't need to lose any more weight. At that point, you would multiply 162 by 14, and you would have your new F14# (daily maximum calorie number).

Now that you have your F14#, what is the best way to structure those calories throughout your day? You will use the 3-2-1 method to prevent plateaus and ensure that you reach your ideal weight. Depending on which plan you select, some days you will have 3 meals, some days 2, and some days 1.

Take your F14# and divide it by 3. This is your maximum calories per meal. This will enable you to eventually make calorie counting seamless because you will know your regular meals by heart, for instance, "I am meeting Edna at Joe Joe's Diner for lunch and know the grilled chicken with corn and green beans equals my 680 calorie meal there., or "Stan and I's favorite meal, a veggie stir fry, is 622 calories."

Now, you will decide on how aggressive you want to be in your journey towards your ideal weight.

Traditional

Day One: 3 meals
Day Two: 3 meals
Day Three: 3 meals
Day Four: 3 meals
Day Five: 3 meals
Day Six: 3 meals
Day Seven: 3 meals

Slow and Steady

Day One: 3 meals
Day Two: 2 meals
Day Three: 3 meals
Day Four: 3 meals
Day Five: 2 meals
Day Six: 3 meals
Day Seven: 3 meals

The Downward Dash

Day One: 3 meals
Day Two: 2 meals
Day Three: 1 meal
Day Four: 1 meal
Day Five: 2 meals
Day Six: 3 meals
Day Seven: 1 meals

The Speed of Sound

Day One: 3 meals
Day Two: 1 meal
Day Three: 3 meals
Day Four: 1 meal
Day Five: 3 meals
Day Six: 1 meal
Day Seven: 2 meals

The Speed of Light

Day One: 3 meals
Day Two: 1 meal
Day Three: 1 meal
Day Four: 1 meal
Day Five: 2 meals
Day Six: 2 meals
Day Seven: 1 meal

Feel free on any given day to have FEWER meals. Also, if you reach a plateau and can't seem to pierce through it, you multiply your ideal weight by 17 and slightly overeat one day per week. Have your last meal at least three hours before bedtime.

So now you have a simple strategy to stay lean forever. For many of you, the journey will end here. "I will just follow this maximum calorie amount for the rest of my life, and it will settle me at or near my ideal weight." I just want to remind you that being thin doesn't necessarily mean you are healthy. It's much healthier than being obese, but there are so many other components that can shift your health in a positive way. I urge you to continue onto the other Formula 14 Phases, where we will address a framework that will keep you on track, nutrition, exercise, and then we begin to address mental and emotional strategies and shift your identity forever.

CHAPTER 2
FORMULA 14 PHASE 2

(HOUR 2/DAY 2/WEEK 2)

THE FORMULA 14 FORGIVENESS FRAMEWORK

I'm a pack mover
I'm a weight loser…

Boss man Dlow

So now you have set your F14 number and plan to never exceed those calories over a 24-hour period for the rest of your life. But what if you do? What if your maximum number of calories is 2000, and you consume 4200? You get back on your F14# the next meal or the next day. This seems like a very simple strategy, but people who struggle with their weight usually don't do this. They think, "Oh no, I broke my diet. Well, I just had a medium pizza, so everything is ruined. I have wanted pancakes for a while now, so I'll see if Tina wants to go to brunch tomorrow. And it's late October with all the kids' yummy Halloween candy, and Thanksgiving is next month, then Christmas. I will get back on this again at New Year's." This leads to months of overeating.

Most people who are overweight forgive themselves for their daily actions that cause weight gain and ill health. Then, the way they look, or a doctor, or a loving friend or family member makes them decide to change things. They decide to go on a diet and exercise plan and bring discipline into their lives. When the diet or exercise plan is broken, and they have a breakdown, they curse themselves and then return to the perpetual state of forgiveness and daily actions that cause weight gain.

So, they are living within a framework that keeps them overweight:

Forgiveness/Discipline framework.

We will flip this and use a Discipline/Forgiveness framework instead. With the Formula 14 DF Framework, we are going to turn this on its head. We will begin the program, be disciplined, adhere to all of the phases, and strive for the ideal: never exceeding the F14 number of calories. The phases you will learn about in later chapters include moving more, an optimal nutrition plan, resistance exercises, proper hydration, what we call an FFT session, etc. When life gets to us and we aren't successful, we will use replacement behaviors to recondition ourselves. If this doesn't work and we break down, we will forgive ourselves immediately and jump back into the program, returning to a state of discipline. This will guide us toward our goals. The DF Discipline/Forgiveness FRAMEWORK:

DISCIPLINE

A disciplined approach to all phases of Formula 14. Some would call it an obsessive approach. Beyond motivation. Motivation can disappear when life knocks you down.

Forget the weak state of having low or no expectations and forgive yourself for horrible food choices and the absence of exercise, etc., on a daily basis.

Set a high standard and live it! Be obsessed with it. But then, if you are about to break down you initially attempt to use the overarching "why" you select later and then the replacement behaviors you will select.

Back to the overall DF framework. Using the F14# as an example, if you are about to eat a pizza and blow your calories, first you would initiate a replacement behavior. Right there in the pizza parlor parking lot, you would close your eyes, do some deep breathing (if that was the chosen replacement behavior), and eventually drive away. If that doesn't work, you contemplate the overarching reason why you are losing weight and see if that outweighs the urge to break down. If none of those steps work and you

BREAKDOWN

and exceed your F14 number of calories, you

FORGIVE

yourself and return to a state of discipline and your F14# of calories the next meal or the next day—not a week later, not a month later, not years, and a 100 lbs weight gain later. Forgive yourself and IMMEDIATELY get back to your F14# maximum daily calories.

So the perpetual state is discipline instead of forgiveness, and your health is much better as you move towards your goals… REGARDLESS OF ANY MINOR SETBACKS!!!

Once I started doing this, it was huge because the old me would start a diet, cut corners, and not really draw a line in the sand. Then, when I realized I had failed, I would say to myself, "Everything is ruined," and begin to overeat and curse myself, saying maybe I will try again next Monday. And it's Wednesday! But when you get a flat tire, do you jump out of the car and flatten the other tires? No! You fix the flat one! If I break down and have a huge dinner with an extra 1500 calories, I can simply forgive myself and then jump right back on it the following morning and still lose weight that week.

So, use Formula 14 to determine your daily calories, and then be rigid and hard on yourself to stay within those calories.

But if you go over, forgive yourself and jump right back on. This is the DF Framework, and if you simply follow your F14 number and make this a rule in your life, you will eventually reach your ideal weight. If you continue and simply add the next phase and design a nutrition plan that works for you long term, you will reach it even quicker!

CHAPTER 3
FORMULA 14 PHASE 3 NUTRITION DUODONICS

(HOUR 3/DAY 3/WEEK 3)

Oh, simple thing, where have you gone?
I'm gettin' old and I need someone to rely on
So, tell me when you're gonna let me in
I'm gettin' tired, and I need somewhere to begin

Somewhere Only We Know - Keane

Now that you have taken charge of overeating with your F14# and committed to the DF Framework, you are ready to take it to the next level and reset your body with vital nutrients. Much of this will depend on your individual tastes and the goals you have for your health. Controlling the quantity of food is one of the most important pieces of the healthy weight loss puzzle. To conquer obesity, any long-term lifestyle nutrition plan must also ultimately address these issues:

1. **Emotional Eating**: Identifying the triggers that make one eat for reasons unrelated to fueling the body, such as filling a lonely void, breaking up a boring daily routine, or escaping stressful situations.

2. **Carbohydrate Addiction**: If a person is addicted to carbohydrates, resolving the issue must begin with their eating strategy. This usually requires a period of low glycemic eating to allow the pancreas to rest and let the taste buds and the entire body adjust. Formula 14 can impact this dramatically, but you may also want to focus on different macros and their impact on your body.

3. **Fuel**: Any long-term eating strategy must provide the body with a steady supply of nutrients to keep the body nourished and the immune system strong.

4. Listen to what your body is telling you and avoid foods that disrupt your energy and health. Is there something you eat that gives you joint pain? Pay attention to the signals your body is sending you, and avoid that food, no matter how much you love the taste! Are you sensitive to certain foods? Dairy and gluten can be a real problem for some people. Don't cause your throat to swell shut like some allergies do (a family friend had a peanut allergy that arose in her 40's), but they can cause inflam-

mation and weight gain. If you sense a problem with a certain food, eliminate it for two weeks and then add it back to see how you feel. There are also tests you can get to identify your problem food. Years ago, I was tested, and they determined that I was allergic to salmon, oranges, crab, and lobster. Meat, dairy, and grains were removed from my diet. My body was flooded with supplementation, veggies, vegetable soup, and a piece of fruit every day. After a week, some nuts were added. Then some avocado. Then brown rice. Eventually, I ate a baked potato three times per week. I started feeling better, and my body began to heal. Consider foods that you eat regularly that seem to bother you.

There are many weight loss programs you can use to lose weight in a safe and effective manner, but first and foremost, the quantity of food one consumes must be addressed. This means ending overeating forever with some form of portion control, which we did in the first phase. Now you must design the best way to eat for you individually that will keep you healthy and thin... by discovering Duodonics, the Delicate Dance Between Protein and Starch for your individual metabolism—the combination that gives you the most energy and allows you to enjoy the healthy foods you love.

This is a personal journey controlled by each individual, your tastes, and your unique metabolism.

FORMULA 14 DUODONICS:

Duodonics is simply finding the best combination of protein and starch for your individual body. The 14 Phases of Duodonics are listed below, and then a detailed description of each will follow:

1. Make the Majority of foods that you consume water-rich.
2. Combine Foods for Energy
3. Reduce or eliminate dairy products from your diet.
4. Reduce meat and fish to 28 small servings (a deck of cards or a smart phone) per month.
5. Reduce eggs to 21 or less per month.
6. Reduce or eliminate refined sugar from your diet.
7. Less alcohol is better, but if you consume it, do not combine it with meals.
8. Make olive oil and avocado your main sources of fat.
9. Reduce or eliminate unhealthy breads and grains.
10. Reduce or eliminate fried foods.
11. Use the Formula 14 Protein Masters Reset.
12. Use the Formula 14 Starch Masters Reset.
13. Use the Formula 14 Fasting Strategies (with your doctor's approval).
14. Use the Formula 14 Muscle Tone Formula.

1. Make the majority of foods you consume water-rich food. What is a water-rich food? A fruit or vegetable that hasn't had its original water content completely cooked out of it. Come up with a list of go-to water-rich foods, keep them on hand, and use them to bolster your consumption with nutrient-dense, energy-giving options. Here is my list of go-to foods: apples, tangerines, grapefruit, strawberries, pineapple, blueberries, cauliflower, broccoli, peas, green beans (especially in green bean casserole—just kidding!), lettuce, various salad greens, avocado, and carrots.

This is not a rigid list, just a group of foods that I know, if I have them on hand, can satisfy cravings and provide my body with nutrients. What about other foods? I believe starch has been given a bad reputation, but it can be an incredible option for many.

For a lean and abundantly healthy body, eat a diet rich in green, living foods (foods that are not processed or overcooked), as well as some nuts and fruits, to help create a strong body with a steady supply of energy. Load lunch and dinner with salad and veggies. For example, if you often eat at a Subway sandwich shop near your work, a salad would be ideal, but if you must have a sandwich, get extra lettuce, tomato, green peppers, and cucumbers. Throw away the top piece of bread and let those living foods energize you, or at least combat some of the effects of the meat and bread. Snack on almonds or raw veggies. Mix it up and have some fun. The more green vegetables you eat, the better. Finding delicious water-rich recipes makes it easy to stick with water-rich foods and be healthier for life!

2. Combine Foods For Energy. Reduce or eliminate meals with both protein and starch. Having steak? Surround it with asparagus. Having a baked potato? Surround it with broccoli. Eat fruit on an empty tummy, first thing in the morning or 3 hours after a regular meal.

3. Reduce or eliminate dairy from your diet. Dairy products are high in fat and cholesterol and contain no fiber— not a wonderful combination.

4. Reduce or eliminate meat and fish from your diet. Get most of your protein from beans and legumes, nuts, and plant-based protein shakes. Beans and legumes are excellent sources of protein for several reasons: They are high in protein, and even though they lack one or more amino acids when paired with grains like rice or wheat, they form a complete protein source, providing all essential amino acids necessary for human health. Beans also have high fiber content and are low in saturated fats but rich in micronutrients. Overall, beans and legumes are

versatile, affordable, and nutrient-dense foods that can be easily incorporated into a balanced diet to meet protein and other nutrient needs. If you do consume meat, fish and, a maximum of 21 servings per month. The serving should be slightly smaller than an average-sized smartphone.

5. Reduce eggs to a maximum of 21 servings per month. Eggs are nutritious and a great source of protein, but limiting egg consumption to 21 per month is recommended for several health reasons, mainly regarding concerns about heart health, cholesterol, and overall dietary balance.

6. Reduce or eliminate refined sugar from your diet. Refined sugar can cause a myriad of dangerous health conditions: obesity, cancer, type two diabetes, and the list goes on and all. Refined sugar has also been linked to mental health challenges and mood swings. Refined sugar can also be so addictive that it can create cycles of cravings and over consumption.

7. Less alcohol is better, but if you drink, do not consume alcohol with meals. Alcohol demands that the liver remove it first, and fat metabolism slows down.

8. Use olive oil and avocado as primary sources of fat. Avocados and olive oil are considered good sources of fats primarily because they contain predominantly monounsaturated fats, which are considered heart-healthy fats. These fats can help lower LDL cholesterol levels (the "bad" cholesterol) and reduce the risk of heart disease when consumed in moderation as part of a balanced diet. Additionally, both avocados and olive oil contain other beneficial nutrients, such as antioxidants and vitamin E, which contribute to their overall health benefits. Other healthy fat sources: nuts and seeds, coconut oil, flaxseeds, chia seeds, grass fed butter and ghee, fatty fish.

9. Reduce or eliminate unhealthy breads and grains. Focus on 100% whole grains and sourdough bread. Reducing or eliminating refined, unhealthy breads and grains in favor of 100% whole grains and sourdough bread can provide numerous health benefits, including better blood sugar control, improved digestion, heart health, and overall nutrient intake. It is a way to increase the quality of your diet while reducing the intake of processed foods that can contribute to chronic diseases.

10. Reduce or eliminate fried foods. Fried foods can be unhealthy for several reasons: they are high in calories, contain trans fats, increase the risk of chronic diseases, are low in nutrients, and can create digestive issues. Overall, while fried foods may be tasty and satisfying, they should be consumed in moderation as part of a balanced diet to minimize their negative health effects. Opting for healthier cooking methods such as baking, grilling, or steaming can help reduce the health risks associated with fried foods.

11. Consider the **Formula 14 Day Protein Masters Reset**

Protein diets can be effective at correcting your metabolism and shedding excess weight. One such eating strategy, the Paleo diet, is derived from the way hunters and gatherers ate two million years ago during the Paleolithic period. The diet consists mainly of meat, fish, and vegetables. Eating grains, dairy, and processed foods is forbidden. Some Paleo advocates also remove fruit until you are lean and healthy. Over the last 10,000 years, human diets have changed to sugar-laden, nutritionally void diets loaded with toxins and chemicals. As a result, we have seen an increase in so many diseases (diabetes, cancer, obesity). Grains are not required for a healthy diet and have been linked to a condition called leaky gut, which affects the lining of the intestines, making you more susceptible to autoimmune disorders. Dairy, famously known to build calcium, is actually shown to do the opposite and may be a cause of osteoporosis. Adding sugar on top of this is just a recipe for disaster. Reverting to the clean way our ancestors ate is one way we can bring our health back into alignment.

Low-carb diets were made famous by Dr. Robert Atkins. Other variations came out later and gave A recent low-carb trend is the Keto Diet. Low-carb dieting usually ends with dramatic weight gain, so what is the upside? It conquers sugar addictions. Because of the fat that you eat freely, you are satiated and feel full. You are not tempting yourself with sugar. I have experienced carbohydrate addiction and know exactly what it is like to have sugar cravings that are almost irresistible. While many people look at those who are obese and judge them harshly, they should realize that natural chemicals in the brain are thousands of times more powerful than the strongest street drugs like cocaine and heroin. When these chemicals are missing, they can make a person reach for sugary foods like an alcoholic reaches for liquor.

On the first morning of a low-carb eating plan, you can have a robust omelet. Even if you consume a large portion of your daily calories, it will trick the brain because of the high protein and fat content. Later in the day, you can eat a salad loaded with grilled chicken, and a low-carb dressing. Anything that breaks a pattern of sugar addiction is an important transitional step. The big problem comes when you tire of the protein and fat and start eating carbs again. If you add back the wrong kinds of carbs, the weight can come roaring back. If you stay within your F14#, you will never have to experience that!

Eat more green vegetables, and you will see some tremendous benefits from low-carb dieting. For your vegetarian or "low-fat" friends who warn you about the dangers of low-carb dieting, remind them: low-carb is better than high sugar/carb, high protein, and high fat! When low-carb dieting, it is not necessary to count the carb grams. Stick to protein and green leafy vegetables, and you can avoid the tedious task of counting carbs, subtracting fiber, and then obsessing over the two remaining carbs you have left at the end of the day. If you are exercising, you may want to add some oatmeal (low sugar) or other low glycemic carbs to give you energy, but that can knock you out of ketosis for a few hours. Ketosis is when there isn't enough glucose from the carbs you eat to provide the body with energy, so fatty acids are released into the bloodstream, converted to ketones, and used for energy to run your body.

The objective here is to remove foods with carbs that are bothersome to your system. By removing them for 14 days, you can determine what foods bother you as you add them back. As far as the list below goes, if there are similar meats and veggie options you enjoy, by all means, eat them for variety. Just use the list and stay within your daily F14#!

FORMULA 14 DAY RESET: PROTEIN MASTERS FOOD LIST

- Beef
- Chicken/Turkey
- Lamb
- Fish/Shellfish
- Nuts (pecan/macadamia/walnut)
- Broccoli
- Cauliflower
- Squash
- Carrots

- Leafy greens
- Avocado
- Tomato
- Peas
- Cucumbers

Use butter/oils sparingly.

After 14 days, begin reintroducing starch to see how your body reacts. The first carbohydrates you reintroduce should be vegetables. When you reintroduce starches, make sure you surround it with vegetables initially and don't mix it with protein. Reintroduce small amounts of fruit on an empty stomach.

12. Consider the **FORMULA 14 Starch Masters Reset.**

You can safely and steadily lose weight on a starch-based diet. Use the list below. You will not be straining your digestive system with meat for two weeks. If you are concerned about getting enough protein, drink plant-based protein shakes. Starch-based does not mean that you should eat bagels, pancakes, and toast all the time. There is new research suggesting that diabetes may result from the massive amount of fat from meat in the bloodstream, which prevents sugar from being removed from the blood and used for energy (Diabetes Care medical journal reference). For now, the objective is to remove foods with proteins that are bothersome to your system. If there are similar starch, fruit, and veggie options you enjoy, by all means, eat them for variety. Just use the list as a guideline and stay within your daily F14#.

Formula 14 Day Reset: Starch Masters Food List

- Sweet/White potatoes
- All rice
- Corn tortillas
- Whole grain or sourdough bread
- Green apples (one per day on an empty stomach)
- Plant-based protein shake (up to 2 daily)
- Broccoli
- Cauliflower
- Squash
- Carrots
- Leafy greens
- Avocado
- Tomato
- Peas
- Cucumbers

Consider B12 supplementation, use butter/oils sparingly, and stay within your F14#.

After 14 days, if desired, begin reintroducing meat/fish to see how your body reacts. The first protein should be eggs, then fish, then other meat. Make sure you surround it with vegetables initially, and don't mix it with starch. If you have a piece of fish or steak, surround it with veggies, not potatoes.

13. Consider intermittent or water-only fasting. **Formula 14 Fasting** utilizes intermittent and water-only fasting to give your digestive system a rest. **Intermittent Fasting.** There are two types of Formula 14 intermittent fasts, which we touched on with the 3-2-1 meal plan in Chapter One: the 6-hour feeding window and the 2-hour feeding window. Regardless of which

feeding window you use, make sure you are not eating within 3 hours of bedtime.

The 6-Hour Feeding Window Formula:
F14# X 0.67 = Total calories over 6 hours (Preferably two meals and/or snacks)

The 2-Hour Feeding Window Formula:
F14# X 0.34 = Total calories over 2 hours

Bouncing between these two formulas is a foolproof strategy for weight loss. Shake it up! If you only have 10 or 15 pounds to lose or are experiencing a plateau, this can get the fat burning off your frame again.

FORMULA 14 WATER-ONLY FASTING

The final option is water-only fasts of 1 to 40 days. Contact Tallis Barker at waterfasting.org if you want to undertake a water-only fast or be under the supervision of your own doctor.

I understand how a water-only fast may seem extreme. I cover this later in more depth on the mental side of weight loss, but there are many diet and exercise programs that people consider extreme: running ultramarathons, climbing mountains, etc. Fasting seems extreme, but there is so much research coming out now that I personally believe can't be denied. Before you cast fasting aside and decide it's not an option for you, research it and discuss it with your Doctor or find a Doctor who is comfortable with the process.

Let me also say that I am not just recommending fasting on a whim. I have successfully completed a 21-day fast, a 30-day fast, and a 40-day fast(specifically a 36-day water fast followed by 4 days of slowly introducing carrot juice). If you decide to fast after talking to your doctor, you will want to do a shorter fast to prove to yourself that you can do it.

Extended water fasting, typically lasting 24 hours or more, has been studied for its potential health benefits, although it's important to note that fasting should be approached with caution and under medical supervision, especially for prolonged durations. Here are some potential benefits supported by peer-reviewed studies:

Weight Loss and Metabolic Health: Research published in Obesity Reviews in 2017 suggests that intermittent fasting, including water fasting, can lead to significant weight loss and improvements in metabolic health markers such as insulin sensitivity and lipid profiles.

Cellular Repair and Autophagy: Fasting triggers autophagy, a process where cells remove damaged components and recycle them for energy. A study published in Cell Metabolism in 2014 found that fasting can induce autophagy in various tissues, potentially promoting cellular repair and longevity.

Inflammation Reduction: Fasting has been shown to reduce inflammation markers in the body. A study published in Cell Research in 2017 demonstrated that fasting can suppress the release of inflammatory cytokines and reduce inflammatory responses in various tissues.

Improved Brain Health: Some studies suggest that fasting may have neuroprotective effects and promote cognitive function. Research published in Cell Metabolism in 2015 indicated that intermittent fasting can enhance synaptic plasticity and protect against age-related cognitive decline in animal models.

Longevity: Although more research is needed in humans, animal studies have shown that caloric restriction, which includes fasting, can extend lifespan. A review published in Cell Metabolism in 2016 summarized evidence from animal studies suggesting that fasting can increase lifespan by promoting metabolic health and reducing oxidative stress.

While these studies suggest the potential benefits of extended water fasting, it's crucial to approach fasting with caution and consider individual health circumstances. Consulting with a healthcare professional before starting a fasting regimen is advisable, especially for individuals with underlying health conditions or those taking medications.

Many people recommend straight fasting to give their digestive systems a rest and to help them lose weight. Others claim a straight fast can throw your body into starvation mode. When the fast ends, you can gain the weight back faster than Violet Beauregarde did at Willy Wonka's Chocolate Factory. For people uncomfortable with the idea of fasting, an abbreviated fast can work wonders.

I believe Fasting can give the body the rest it needs to heal itself. In terms of being healthy and detoxifying, there are powerful arguments for fasting. Were our digestive systems designed to handle the huge amounts of food we eat throughout the day, or could this system use some occasional rest? Waterfasting.org is an incredible resource, and Dr. Tallis Barker has guided hundreds of people through successful fasts.

Ultimately, make quantity control fun and don't go to extremes. Fasting should be used to address major health issues and be supervised by a doctor, and ultimately return to normal consumption.

14. Consider the muscle tone formula if you are working to add muscle. FORMULA 14 Muscle Tone Formula

Inevitably, when you start a new eating pattern or exercise plan, you will be asked, "Where do you get your protein?" With the Formula 14 Muscle Tone Formula, you get plenty! The Formula 14 strategy for building or preserving lean muscle mass is to eat 14 grams of protein for every 16 pounds of ideal body weight. Here is Formula 14 for Muscle Mass:

IDEAL BODY WEIGHT / 16 = ______ X 14 = DAILY PROTEIN REQUIREMENT

Once you have determined your daily protein requirement, multiply it by 4. This is the number of daily calories you will dedicate to protein. The remaining calories can be used as you wish, remembering that fruits and veggies are healthier than fast food and candy. This doesn't mean that you can't indulge in richer foods and treats you like, especially in the one-hour window after a tough workout in the gym when your body will use these foods differently. Here is an example of Formula 14 for Muscle Mass using a person with an ideal weight of 200 lbs:

200 / 16 = 12.5 x 14 = 175 grams of protein. 175 x 4 = 700 calories of protein daily. This would leave the person with 2100 calories daily for fat and carbs.

If you are working out but not getting the gains you want, increase the protein to a larger percentage of your daily diet. "How in the hell can I get that much protein?" you groan. "Especially if I want to be vegetarian?" your cousin moans. If you are already eating processed foods, a Zone Bar has 14 grams of protein. Have a couple. What about a delicious piece of tilapia? A 3.5-ounce serving contains 26 grams of protein! Also, remember that other foods will provide some protein, so don't forget many plant-based options with protein shakes, etc. Don't let this overwhelm you.

If you like to eat beef and chicken as your primary source of protein, consider this: cows and chickens have warmer body temperatures than humans, so their fat becomes thicker and stickier in our bloodstreams. Fish are different because they are cold-blooded, so their fat liquefies in the human bloodstream. So, when you can, choose fish over chicken and beef, provided it doesn't come from a mercury-laden source.

THE DIET OF YOUR CHOICE

Nutrition dominates most weight loss books, usually leaving emotional and mental strategies for you to figure out. My approach is different. If you are following Formula 14 to control your intake and quantity, staying properly hydrated, exercising, and using supplementation (described in greater detail in a later phase) wisely, then almost any diet you pick will give you good weight loss results. I want to reiterate that weight loss and health are not always the same thing, but almost any diet and exercise plan with supplementation and enough water is better than overeating toxic and fatty foods.

There are so many diets to pick from: Is Weight Watchers™ your favorite diet? Jump on the point system. You will be addressing two major components of being healthy: overconsumption and proper hydration. Is keto or low-carb your cup of tea? Follow the plan as long as you can, and then fall back on

Formula 14 and keep your intake below your F14#, and the fat will keep melting away. One word of warning when combining the diet of your choice: diet sodas, excess protein consumption, and many other factors will create an acidic environment in your body. This can slow down the rate of your weight loss. If that happens, make sure you add more living foods to your diet, not eating more than your Formula 14 maximum amount of daily calories, and you will begin losing weight again.

The diet of choice for some people is no diet at all. You've probably heard that really all you need to do is to eat sensibly and exercise. Some people do require guidance and structure, but it isn't necessary for those with good willpower. This reminds me of a story a friend of mine told me. His doctor commented on some of his blood work and his 30 extra pounds and told him he needed to lose weight. My friend asked his doctor, "What do I need to do?" He expected his doctor to provide him with a list of foods or to recommend a specific diet and exercise plan. His doctor smiled and simply said, "You know what to do." We all know steps that we can take to improve our health and things we can eliminate that damage our health. Arnold Schwarzenegger once said he heard someone talk about needing to lose a little weight and how hard it was and thought to himself, "I would hate myself if I was that weak." If we all had the weight loss discipline of Arnold, we would not rely on the latest weight loss drugs, hormone injections, and fad diets. Instead, we would intuitively know what consumption and exercise strategies we needed.

I often find myself in patterns of eating where I have the same breakfast, lunch, and dinner for weeks at a time. The body adapts to certain food choices, and variety can be very helpful in providing the body with different nutrients. Mixing it up also gives the mind some variety that can keep you on a path toward weight loss.

If you have a diet that is practical and easier to follow, couple it with the other Formula 14 strategies in this book. It can make you lean and create high levels of energy throughout the day.

A final word on nutrition: Our discussion here focused on weight loss. There are other compelling reasons to shift your consumption patterns. Heart disease, diabetes, and cancer are just a few. So, when you are looking for the best eating strategy for you, make sure you consider your health as well. Diets do work. It has become a cute phrase in health and fitness circles now to say, "Diets don't work. You have to change your lifestyle and eat healthier." Or, the first three letters in the word diet are DIE. But any temporary change is going to be just that: temporary. But don't use that as an excuse to overeat whatever you want by sighing and saying, "Diets just don't work." Diets work, if you never quit dieting. And with Formula 14, you always have your F14# to fall back on to block obesity and overconsumption so you can be successful.

Example: Tammy spends two months on a Keto diet but is getting tired of the carb restriction. She is getting restless and knows she is about to break down, so she switches to Weight Watchers and finds more variety and the added benefit of meeting with others who are also serious about losing weight. Six months later, she gets tired of the meetings, and her weight loss plateaus, so she orders Nutrisystem™ to be delivered to her home for convenience. By shifting from diet to diet for three years, she loses 214 pounds. Now, at this point, if she starts eating like she did when she was obese, then, of course, the weight will come surging back. That goes without saying. Tammy was just on a series of diets—and she never gained the weight back. Now, she is 214 lbs. thinner and can focus on the healthiest eating system for her body. Food for thought.

So, to sum up, Formula 14 Nutrition: find a path that suits your tastes and your ability to follow through, always being cognizant of your F14# and not overeating. You always have that to fall back on.

CHAPTER 4
FORMULA 14 PHASE 4
(HOUR 4/DAY 4/WEEK 4)

DESIGN YOUR EXERCISE

There is Joy in Repetition

Prince

Let me start this chapter with another disclaimer. Before starting any exercise program, check with your doctor. Get probed, prodded, and then pressured by your doctor to undertake a new exercise program, and then return to this chapter. Did you get that check-up? I didn't think so. Read the chapter and then schedule it!

Most people would be amazed at what their bodies could accomplish right now. Stu Mittleman is an ultra-distance runner who ran 1,000 miles in just over 11 days. That is three marathons a day! In his book *Slow Burn,* Mittleman says people can do more than they think they can. According to Stu, "we need to stretch beyond self-imposed limitations." He was hired as a consultant to prepare a team of runners for the New York City Marathon. The problem was that most of the 27 runners had only run in 5k races, and only one of them had run a full marathon. Mittleman only had nine weeks to train the team to run. So, he told them they were going to learn how to participate in a "26.2-mile street festival." Every aid station was going to be a festival booth where the team would quench their thirst and rejoice. All of the runners completed the marathon, and one of them even said, "I will never doubt myself again." [1]

So, if you have not exercised in a long time, do not be discouraged. You will not have to run a marathon in nine weeks; you can pick an exercise that you like and figure out a way to make it fun and enjoyable.

First, let's talk about creating an aerobic exercise plan that is tailored to your lifestyle. Increasing your aerobic capacity will

---

1. Mittleman, Stu, Slow Burn, Harper Collins, 2000, pp 3-7

train your metabolism to choose fat as its primary source of fuel.

AEROBIC EXERCISE

Aerobic means "with oxygen." When you are exercising in an aerobic state, your breathing should be steady and deep, not labored. Aerobic exercise is the foundation of any exercise program. To find your target heart rate zones, subtract your age from 220, then multiply by 60%. This is the heartbeats per minute for the bottom end of your target range. Multiply by 90% to get the top end of your target zone. The formula for a forty-year-old person would look like this: 220 - 40 x .60 = 108 beats per minute, 220 - 40 x .90 = 162 beats per minute. So, the target zone for aerobic exercise would be 108 to 162 beats per minute.

That is just a formula for the average person to use as a guide. If you don't have a heart rate monitor or a professional who can test you to give you accurate heart rate target zones, simply make sure that you are slightly winded but can still carry on a conversation. If you can talk easily without ever having to catch your breath, then you are probably not working hard enough. Most treadmill and elliptical machines now have sensors you can grasp, and the machine will give you your heart rate. Create a strong aerobic foundation, and when you jump up from the couch to grab a glass of water, your body will choose more fat as fuel and less glycogen.

The goal is to build to a minimum of 5 weekly sessions of 40 minutes of aerobic exercise. This is a minimum, and as you move towards an hour or more daily, your aerobic capacity will continue to improve.

MORE MOVEMENT

Another option to burn calories and increase your conditioning is simply to fidget and move around more. When you stream a show, stand up and move. When you go to the grocery store, move around the store briskly. Tense muscles all over your body when you are sitting at your desk and talking to clients. You will be stunned at how effective this can be at making you leaner over time.

Another system you can use is to monitor your daily steps and use your smartphone to see what you have been averaging lately. If it's 2,600 per day, start walking more and increasing it. Your ultimate goal will be 7000 to 14,000 steps per day, at least 5 days per week.

Finally, how can you move more in your daily life? I used to call upstairs and ask one of the kids to bring down my charger or whatever I needed because I was too lazy to walk up the stairs and get it myself. If you are on a weekend getaway and the weather permits, walk 10 minutes to the restaurant you are having your next meal at instead of driving. Also, sprinkle the trip with physical activities if you aren't normally inclined to do so.

RESISTANCE EXERCISE

FREE HAND EXERCISES

You can use free hand exercises, weights, or a combination of the two to tone your body. There is something fascinating about free-hand exercises because they can be done anywhere. My brother Jay developed a system to tone his muscles while sitting at his desk or in the middle of traffic. He turned his forearms into bulging slabs of steel that would make Popeye proud, all while sitting in the car or at his office. When challenged by a professional arm wrestling champion, Jay reluctantly agreed to take him on and was stunned at how easy it was to beat him. I am amazed by the size of my brother's arms, and he developed them sitting in a chair watching TV or working. Jay worked on different moves over and over, honing his muscle contraction exercises, and a new method for building the body was created: Flexaholics.

I like to do a combination of free hand exercises and high repetitions with a light weight at home. This is the system that I used to get lean, and my coaching clients love how simple and convenient it is. Go to formula14hometone.com for videos on how to complete each exercise:

THE FORMULA 14 HOME TONE EXERCISE PLAN:

Day 1: Arms and Back
One Arm Dumbbell Row Side Grip
One Arm Dumbbell Row Forward Grip
Two Arm Dumbbell Row Side Grip
Standing Alternate Dumbbell Curl

Standing Two Arm Hammer Curls
Concentration Curls
Forearm dumbbell curls
Forearm Reverse Dumbbell Curls

Day 2: Shoulders and Abs
Dumbbell Shoulder Press
Lateral Deltiod Dumbbell Raises
Bent Over Rear Deltiod Dumbbell Raises
Front Deltoid Shoulder Raises
Crunches: Middle, Left, Right
Knee Raises

Day 3: Chest and Triceps
Push-Ups
Diamond Push-Ups
Wide Push-Ups
One-Arm Dumbbell Triceps Extension (Lying Down)
Overhead Triceps Extension (both hands one dumbbell)
Chair Dips

Day 4; Legs and Abs
Chair squats
Calf Raises
Crunches: Middle, Left, Right
Knee Raises

I like to do a free hand session early in the morning or right before bed. I start with some jumping jacks to get the blood flowing, then do the Formula 14 Home Tone exercises. Don't get overwhelmed and put it off if some of the exercises are too hard in the beginning. Just do easier variations and build up. With all the push-up exercises, I am embarrassed to say I started standing up against the wall! I started with a few reps and then added reps every time I worked my chest. Eventually, I moved to the floor and was getting a great workout. I told my brother and a friend about this. We all got a good laugh when my brother asked, "Did you clap in between each rep like they do in the military?"

Make your resistance exercises fun, and start slow if needed. There are so many great books and variations to choose from. Like I mentioned before, I started my push-up quest with 10 push-ups standing and leaning into the wall. Then I moved to 12, eventually ending up on the floor doing them correctly.

FREE WEIGHTS/NAUTILUS

For those of you who love going to the gym or want increased muscle mass, you can use free weights and other exercise machines. With free weights, you can target specific muscles, get a good "burn" or contraction, and then rest the muscle for a few days while it grows.

There are basic exercises that you can use to target each designated area of the body. I will list a few here, and you can see how the exercises are performed on YouTube or, better yet, hire a personal trainer to teach you basic form. The exercises are: the squat, the lunge, the chest press, the chest fly, the pull-down, the row, the shoulder press, side raises, the press down, the extension, the curl, the crunch, and the reverse crunch.

The objective is to shock the muscles while avoiding overworking them. For example, if you have been doing standing dumbbell curls, you might want to sit on a bench in a reclined position to target the biceps better. The less your muscles are allowed to adapt, the more they will grow. The more muscle mass in your body, the faster your metabolism....

Some additional training suggestions:

Get plenty of sleep every night. The muscles must be allowed to recuperate. When you are targeting your muscles intensely (especially if a personal trainer is taking them to "failure"), they must get enough rest.

Focus your full attention on the muscle that you are working. Block out all distractions as you work through the range of motion. This will speed up your progress.

NEGATION TENSION

New research suggests that slowing down the negative progression when you are doing toning exercises can dramatically increase the muscle you build. For example, when you do a push-up, start on the floor and push up at the traditional speed. When you go back towards the floor, slow it down dramatically. Pushing up takes a second, while lowering yourself back to the floor takes 60 seconds. This can be done with a series of exercises. For calf raises, burst upward, then slowly lower your body. For squats, burst upward, then slowly collapse into the squat. This tears the muscle down, and you will be shocked at how quickly you tone.

COMBINATION TRAINING

Combining aerobic and anaerobic exercise can also help you lose dramatic amounts of weight quickly. Once you have established a fat-burning metabolism with aerobic exercise, you can mix in short bursts of anaerobic exercise to accomplish your weight loss goals faster. Adjust the speeds and the incline on the treadmill in three-minute cycles. Bounce from push-ups and squats to a few sprints. Mix it up and have fun!

STRETCHING

A good stretching routine helps improve flexibility, reduce muscle tension, and enhance overall performance. Here's a simple, effective routine you can follow:

Pre-Stretch Warm-Up (5 minutes)
Jog in place or jump rope: 2-3 minutes to increase blood flow and warm up muscles.
Arm circles and leg swings: 1-2 minutes to loosen joints and prepare for stretching.

Stretching Routine (10-15 minutes)
1. **Neck Stretch:** Gently tilt your head to each side, holding for 15-20 seconds. Repeat on each side.
2. **Shoulder Stretch:** Bring one arm across your body and hold with the opposite hand for 20-30 seconds. Repeat on the other side.
3. **Triceps Stretch:** Raise one arm overhead, bend the elbow,

and use the opposite hand to push down gently. Hold for 20-30 seconds each side.

4. **Chest Stretch:** Stand in a doorway, place your hands on the frame, and gently lean forward. Hold for 20-30 seconds.
5. **Side Stretch:** Reach one arm overhead and bend to the opposite side. Hold for 20-30 seconds each side.
6. **Quad Stretch:** Stand on one leg, pull the opposite foot toward your buttocks, and hold for 20-30 seconds. Use a wall for balance if needed. Repeat on the other side.
7. **Hamstring Stretch:** Sit on the ground with one leg extended, reach for your toes, and hold for 20-30 seconds. Repeat with the other leg.
8. **Calf Stretch:** Stand facing a wall, place one foot behind you, and press the heel into the ground. Hold for 20-30 seconds each leg.
9. **Hip Flexor Stretch:** Kneel on one knee, push your hips forward, and hold for 20-30 seconds. Repeat on the other side.
10. **Child's Pose:** Sit back on your heels, extend your arms forward, and lower your chest to the ground. Hold for 30 seconds.

Post-Stretch Cool Down (2-3 minutes)

Deep Breathing: Focus on slow, deep breaths to help your body relax.

Light Walking: Walk around to gradually bring your heart rate down.

This routine can be performed daily or after workouts to maintain flexibility and reduce the risk of injury.

Exercise is important, but make sure you don't overdo it. This can actually slow down your weight loss by creating excess acid in the body. Ultimately, an exercise plan needs to be interesting, challenging, and fun. If getting down on the floor and doing free hand exercises during a break at the office is unimaginable to you, then stick with a thirty-minute morning run through the park and your circuit training at the gym. If the thought of getting dressed up and going to the gym is dreadful and draining to you, then jump on your treadmill or exercise bike and get busy! Action is the key, so take the famous advice from yesteryear and Nike™ and JUST DO IT!

Oftentimes, the moment requires good old-fashioned action. No planning, no strategizing; just action. Successful people in any endeavor usually contemplate, plan, and are decisive. When the time comes, they dive in headfirst to get things done. They take action and get moving BEFORE THEY ARE READY. They understand conditions will never be perfect. They know they must act to get things done. Be one of these people starting right now.

What really works for you is all that matters. You have to find the strategies that propel you forward and the things that hold you back. With Formula 14, there is a strategy you can craft from the previous pages that will work for you. Your task now is to determine what that is and get started on your journey, creating the healthy lifestyle that you desire.

When it comes to building muscle and toning the body, a personal trainer can also be helpful because they hold you accountable and know various exercises to keep it interesting and continue shocking your muscles. A good personal trainer has a deep knowledge of the body and its systems and can safely push you. When I first started working out, I was scared to push myself. Once, I complained that my knee was a little sore, and my trainer said, “Did you get your wife to rub it?” He was not letting me off that easy. The human body is resilient and can be pushed more than we think. Whenever I start whining in the gym, I think of the power of the human body and its ability to survive and thrive.

Think about the training required to become a Navy SEAL. You must endure Hell Week, a five-day endeavor where you get to sleep for a whopping total of four hours. When you are awake, you run up and down the beach carrying logs and rubber rafts filled with water. You have to endure "surf torture," running in and out of the freezing surf, your body pushed to the edge of hypothermia. By the end of Hell Week, the participants sleep for almost 24 hours straight and are so exhausted that they have to be monitored by other soldiers because an arm hanging off the edge of a bed can become so swollen with fluids.

When I think of the incredible power of the human body, I also think of Beck Weathers. Weathers survived for more than 24 hours in sub-zero weather and brutal winds on Mount Everest. He was comatose for 12 hours, and parts of his hand and face were frozen. Something stirred deep within, and he woke up and stumbled for ninety minutes down to the camp.

While I am on the subject of the human body enduring much more than we think it can, a few years back, I saw a movie called *127 Hours*. This is the true story of Aaron Ralston, an outdoor enthusiast, who was hiking, and his arm became pinned to a canyon wall by a giant rock. After being stuck for five days, he acknowledged the unthinkable. The only way he was going to survive was to amputate his own arm and hike back to his car. He tied a tourniquet around his arm, broke the bone, and used a dull utility knife to cut his arm off. He then walked for miles, even rappelled down a cliff, until he ran into some hikers and was airlifted to a nearby hospital.

Now, I am not suggesting that you join the Navy SEALs, get stranded on the face of Mount Everest, or amputate your own arm. These are three extreme examples, but they do inspire me to reach deeper when I am whining about how hard a workout or an eating regimen is. And remember, even if the body can endure a tremendous amount of stress and be pushed beyond its limits, it doesn't mean it has to be, especially if it compromises your health! This would probably be a good point to give you another disclaimer: I am not an exercise physiologist or personal trainer, so make sure you get a doctor's approval before you begin any exercise program!

Now that you have discovered your F14#, embraced the Forgiveness Framework, Designed your nutritional plan, and designed an exercise plan you can stick with consistently, let's dive into Section Two to bolster vitality and continue the journey to losing weight and being healthy.

SECTION TWO

THE FABULOUS FIVE

5. Supreme Hydration
6. Supplementation
7. Sleep, Rest
8. Stress Busting
9. Breathing

CHAPTER 5
FORMULA 14 PHASE 5

(HOUR 5/DAY 5/WEEK 5)

FORMULA 14 OZ OF WATER, HYDRATION

There is freedom within, there is freedom without
Try to catch a deluge in a paper cup
There's a battle ahead, many battles are lost
But you'll never see the end of the road
While you're traveling with me

Hey now, hey now, don't dream it's over
Hey now, hey now, when the world comes in
They come, they come to build a wall between us
We know they won't win

Don't dream it's over - Crowded House

FORMULA 14 AND SUPREME HYDRATION

After air, water is the most critical element for our survival. Stop drinking water for a few days, and you can experience severe health challenges. Many Americans are dehydrated, and overweight people are often chronically dehydrated. To get the proper amount of water, drink a minimum of five 14 oz servings of water daily. A little wine or coffee is okay, but do your best to avoid sugary drinks whenever possible. There is a specific water I have consumed that I believe is the best water in the world, and I believe you should consume it instead of bottled, tap, or other filtered water. Go to formula14water.com for more information.

Now that you are happily hydrated, let's consider supplementation:

CHAPTER 6
FORMULA 14 PHASE 6

(HOUR 6/DAY 6/WEEK 6)

DESIGN YOUR SUPPLEMENTATION

So I pause a second, acknowledging a cheap thrill
Was the cause of this mammoth thick bitter pill
Ha-I'm laughing now
Surprise! I'm smiling still
Full Fruition

Full Fruition - Barbaree Church

I believe supplementation is important, but there are so many wild claims about products that it makes it hard to determine which supplements are best. A deficiency in certain nutrients may not be obvious to you. Often, they are subclinical and will simply drain your energy and lead to more serious problems down the road. That being said, many supplements use unhealthy fillers, and in hospitals, they are known as "bedpan bullets" because they don't break down properly. Do your research and find a reputable company for your supplements. Here is a list of supplements I have found useful:

SUPPLEMENTS FOR WEIGHT LOSS AND GENERAL WELL-BEING

1. **A Good Multivitamin**: Many of our foods are devitalized these days, so it is important to ensure that your body is receiving the basic nutrients it needs to be healthy.

2. **Omega-3 Fatty Acids**: These are essential and not made by the body, so they must come from supplements or through the daily diet. Omega-3s may seriously lower the risks associated with heart disease and reduce levels of homocysteine in the blood, which has been linked to heart disease, stroke, Alzheimer's, and Parkinson's disease. They can also act as blood thinners, preventing clots and reducing the risk of heart attacks.

3. **Turmeric**: The main spice in curry, turmeric is popular for its anti-inflammatory properties and other health benefits. A family member with undifferentiated connective tissue disorder and immune deficiency found relief with turmeric when other treatments failed. I took 600 mg of turmeric and 50 mg of turmeric oil almost every morning for years, and I believe it may have prevented serious medical events while I was overweight.

Ensure you get the purest form available, manufactured in a facility dedicated to turmeric supplementation.

4. **Digestive Enzymes**: These help assimilate your food when your body is low on reserves. There are 14 different enzymes, so find a supplement with as many as possible.

5. **Coenzyme Q-10**: Required for cellular energy, CoQ-10 is involved in the creation of ATP, the foundation of energy throughout the body. It improves energy function and acts as an antioxidant, which may help fight heart disease and cancer.

6. **GABA**: A brain chemical similar to Valium, but available without a prescription, GABA can have a calming effect and help you relax.

7. **L-Glutamine**: An amino acid that helps conquer sugar cravings, L-glutamine can support brain chemistry and keep your mind sharp. It's also beneficial for those with intestinal permeability (Leaky Gut Syndrome), a condition now recognized as real by new studies.

8. **Chromium**: This mineral can help balance blood sugar and curb sugar cravings. Your multivitamin should provide an adequate amount.

9. **Green Drinks and Herbal Supplements**: These can help cleanse and alkalize your body, especially if you dislike green vegetables. They offer nutrients and cleansing properties and are a good option for those with a history of heavy meat consumption.

10. A zeolite compound that can penetrate the cell wall and help your body remove heavy metals and other toxins.

THE IMPORTANCE OF CLEANSING

How do you know if you need a cleanse? Symptoms include constant fatigue, a history of antibiotic use, obesity, body odor or bad breath, poor complexion, and difficulty with bowel movements. Various cleansing options are available, from cellular cleanses to colon cleanses. Effective colon cleansing systems should include psyllium, montmorillonite clay, and herbs like butternut root bark, cascara sagrada bark, rhubarb root, ginger root, licorice root, Irish moss, and cayenne.

There are many other supplements available that may be helpful. Exotic juices and other supplements are worth testing if you do your research or know someone who has had success. However, avoid the trap of thinking a miracle supplement will allow you to eat whatever you want and still lose weight. Your weight loss strategy should have a solid foundation, and while supplementation may be a part of it, it is never the end-all-be-all.

CHAPTER 7
FORMULA 14 PHASE 7

(HOUR 7/DAY 7/WEEK 7)

FORMULA 14 DEEP SLEEP, REST

She told me
"A bit of madness is key
To give us new colors to see
Who knows where it will lead us?
And that's why they need us"
So bring on the rebels
The ripples from pebbles
The painters, and poets, and plays
And here's to the fools who dream
Crazy as they may seem
Here's to the hearts that break
Here's to the mess we make

Audition - La La Land

REST AND SLEEP

The importance of nerve energy cannot be overstated. The human body operates like a series of wires with electrical pulses surging through them. These electrical pulses send signals at the most basic level for cells to thrive and must have sufficient electrical power. What could disrupt this? We previously discussed how charges around red blood cells can be affected. Additionally, challenges within the spinal column can cause the electrical pulses to fire more slowly. Factors like cell phones, computer screens, and even staring into a microwave to check if the soup is hot enough can have an impact. Wi-Fi signals also play a role. It might seem overwhelming to worry about all these factors, but why not attempt to prevent some of the damage that today's lifestyles and technology might cause? Proper breathing, exercise, sleep, and rest can help your body cope. This will increase your energy levels, prepare your body to battle the "bugs" that come around every winter, and deflect some of the stress and strain that today's society can place on your body.

People are busy in today's fast-paced society, so ensure that your body has the energy it needs by getting proper sleep and relaxation. This area is a constant struggle for me. I love to stay up in the evenings. Some people flourish with quick naps throughout the day. You can also take a simple sensory rest by going to a quiet place, closing your eyes, and relaxing for a few minutes.

When it comes to actually sleeping, make sure you follow the four Golden Rules of Sleep created by Dr. James Maas:

1. Get an adequate amount of sleep every night.
2. Establish a regular sleep schedule.
3. Get continuous sleep.
4. Make up for lost sleep. [1]

An adequate amount of sleep is whatever it takes to remain alert throughout the day. For most people, this is 7 or 8 hours; some people can get by on a little less, and others need a little more. As we discussed in the exercise section, you will require more sleep if your muscles have worked hard and need time to rejuvenate and rebuild. A regular sleep schedule is one that allows you to go to bed at the same time at night and wake up at the same time every morning, without an alarm clock, 7 days a week. One continuous block of sleep is always better than broken sleep, and if you do have to pull an all-nighter, make sure you make up those hours as soon as possible by returning to your established sleep schedule.

1. Maas, Dr. James B., Power Sleep, Quill, 1998, pg. 71

CHAPTER 8
FORMULA 14 PHASE 8
(HOUR 8/DAY 8/WEEK 8)

STRESS BUSTING WITH FORMULA 14 FLIGHT, FIGHT OR THRIVE SESSIONS

Does it feel that your life's become a catastrophe?
Oh, it has to be, for you to grow boy
When you look through the years and see what you could have been
Oh, what you might have been
If you would have had more time

Take the Long Way Home - Supertramp

Stress can have an intense physiological impact on your body. When something stressful happens, the body is flooded with cortisol. Insulin is released to counteract the cortisol, making stress akin to eating a king-sized Butterfinger™. Insulin causes fat storage, and a stressful life creates a cycle of weight gain and serious health challenges.

Many people allow stress to build up until they scream at the people they love. The tension needs to be released, and you can do it in a way that empowers you and doesn't negatively impact those you care about (or even strangers in traffic).

Nature can have a calming effect on people. The beach and the mountains are ideal places to recharge your batteries and relax. Environmental stress from the hustle and bustle of city life can be unhealthy, and weekend getaways can energize and revitalize your soul.

Meditation is a powerful way to relieve stress. Dr. Dean Ornish uses it in his program, that has reversed heart disease in some patients. Meditation is a personal endeavor, and each individual must find a path that is comfortable. Find a system that you are comfortable with, even if it's just sitting quietly for a few minutes at a time.

Get control of your stress triggers, and you will be stunned at how it renders the tension powerless. This can help you avoid a total free fall and a binge day, or a new series of "last suppers." The most important mindset is to forgive yourself quickly and jump back on the path, as we discussed with the Formula 14 Forgiveness Framework.

Three daily Formula 14 Minute Stress Buster Sessions will

help condition you to handle stressful situations more easily. These sessions will help pull you out of fight or flight mode and allow you to calmly draw on more resourceful states to battle stress.

Sit quietly and make sure you are in touch with one of your five senses. I learned how to do this from Shirzad Chamine, who wrote a powerful book called Positive Intelligence. His research shows that when you are in fight or flight mode, your body shuts down and focuses on one task, like getting away from a bear you encounter while hiking. If you focus on one of the five senses with your eyes closed, it puts you into a calm state of resourcefulness that you can use in stressful situations. One example Chamine suggests is listening to the furthest away sound you can hear, then bringing it closer and listening to yourself breathe. If you were running from a bear, you wouldn't be able to contemplate the sounds you were hearing in your environment; you would have to focus on the path ahead and run like hell.

Although I used the example of a bear, your survival brain doesn't know the difference between a bear running at you, your boss telling you you have a massive project due in two days, or your boyfriend telling you he is sitting down to have lunch with your husband in five minutes and is going to tell him everything.

Another path to reach this state is to become much more aware of your surroundings in your day-to-day life. Eckhart Tolle, who wrote the international best seller The Power of Now, says:

"In your everyday life, you can practice this by taking any routine activity that normally is only a means to an end, and giving it your fullest

attention, so that it becomes an end in itself. For example, every time you walk up and down the stairs in your house or place of work, pay close attention to every step, every movement, even your breathing. Be totally present. Or when you wash your hands, pay attention to all the sense perceptions associated with the activity: the sound and feel of the water, the movement of your hands, the scent of the soap, and so on. Or when you get into your car, after you close the door, pause for a few seconds, and observe the flow of your breath. Become aware of a silent, but powerful sense of presence. There is one certain criterion by which you can measure your success in this practice: the degree of peace that you feel within." [1]

He describes this activity as a path to enlightenment, and on the way there, it will also provide you with the means of escaping the fight or flight stresses of life by tuning into one of the five senses.

The goal is to create a 14-minute Fight, Flight, or Thrive session for yourself, where you close your eyes and purposefully get into a state where you notice one of your five senses, or do what Tolle suggests and accomplish it in your day-to-day life. When you walk across the parking lot into work, notice the different colors of the cars or listen to all the sounds in your environment (something you could never do if Michael Myers stepped from behind a car with a large butcher knife—you would be running and focused on one thing: getting out of there!).

Ultimately, you want to build to three 14-minute sessions daily, or a combination of 42 minutes of stress-busting to equip yourself to deal with the stresses of life.

With all of these phases of Formula 14, you know what to do

---

1. Tolle, Eckhart, Practicing the Power of Now,1999, pg. 21-22.

to lose weight; you simply need to take action on what you know and not let stress derail you. The majority of the battle is the mental struggle. When a person decides to quit smoking, they can quit cold turkey and never look back. You can't stop eating, so it is a much more difficult challenge. We all have a lifetime of pleasurable experiences eating with friends and family. These positive experiences are hardwired through neural pathways and are linked to our decisions. We are also bombarded with hundreds of external messages every day. The fast food giants spend hundreds of millions of dollars to sell us their products. Ultimately, we have to take charge of our own lives.

CHAPTER 9

FORMULA 14 PHASE 9

(HOUR 9/DAY 9/WEEK 9)

FORMULA 14 BREATHING EXERCISES

Bound in a nutshell
Lost in our weary eyes
We're tumbledown people
Leading our tumbledown lives
Breath of life (breath of life)
Could make our engines roar
Oh we're far from power, north of desire
High and dry, hoping you'll send us
From your mouth instead of lies
A kiss of life for sleeping giants

Bound in a Nutshell - The Lightening Seeds

DEEP BREATHING EXERCISES:

Your blood has a pump (the heart) that moves it around through your body. However, your lymph system, which removes dead cells and other toxins, can only be stimulated by deep breathing and movement. Taking deep lymphatic breaths is the best way to stimulate the flow of lymph in the body. Breathing in a 1-4-2 ratio is the best way to oxygenate the bloodstream and stimulate the flow of lymph. So, if you were to inhale through the nose for 4 seconds, you would hold for 16 seconds and exhale through the mouth for 8 seconds. If you inhaled for 2 seconds you would hold for 8 and exhale for 4 seconds, etc. Do at least 14 of these lymphatic breaths every day.

ALTERNATING NOSTRIL BREATHING EXERCISES

There is another breathing exercise that can calm you and balance out your nervous system. Sit down and take a deep breath through your nose, and exhale through your mouth. Then, use a finger to block your right nostril and inhale through your left nostril for a count of six. Hold the breath for a count of three, then block your left nostril and release the air through the right nostril. Exhale for a count of six out of the right nostril. Take a deep breath and then reverse the process, beginning with your left nostril blocked. Do at least 14 daily repetitions, and you will feel the balancing effect.

The breath should be smooth and even, avoiding any strain or force. Practicing this technique regularly can help reduce stress and anxiety, improve cardiovascular function, and enhance overall lung capacity.

In addition to its calming effects, alternate nostril breathing can also enhance cognitive function and improve focus. This practice can increase oxygenation and balance the activity between the brain's hemispheres, potentially leading to improved mental performance and a heightened sense of well-being. By integrating alternate nostril breathing into your daily routine, you can experience its myriad benefits, promoting a harmonious balance between mind, body, and spirit.

Breathing in the 1-4-2 ratio and alternate nostril breathing benefit overall bodily functions, including oxygenation and lymph fluid movement, which can aid your journey to your ideal weight!

CALMING BREATHS

Double inhale through the nose. The first one is a complete inhale so your lungs feel full. Then you sneak in a little more air with a second inhale through the nose. Then, a long, slow exhale with the mouth.

SECTION THREE

THE FINAL FIVE: A TOTAL IDENTITY SHIFT

10. Identity Shift Part One (what I gain from being overweight, 14 reasons why, the overarching reason

11. Identity Shift Part Two: 14 Replacement Behaviors, The Two Paths Meditation

12. Identity Shift Part Three: Your Magnificent Event, External Forces, The Lords of Discipline, The Extremes, The Tortoise and the Hare

13. Identity Shift Part Four: Power Phrasing

14. Identity Shift Part Five: Aligning your Words and Actions, Taking Total Responsibility, The Self Integrity Snowball

CHAPTER 10
FORMULA 14 PHASE 10
(HOUR 10/DAY 10/WEEK 10)

IDENTITY SHIFT PART ONE. WHAT DO I GAIN FROM BEING OVERWEIGHT?, 14 REASONS WHY, THE OVERARCHING REASON

I stood in the unsheltered place
'Til I could see the face behind the face
All that had gone before had left no trace

Down by the railway siding
In our secret world we were colliding
All the places we were hiding love
What was it we were thinking of?

Peter Gabriel - Secret World

When it comes to weight loss and your health, your emotions play a key role in accomplishing your goals. To make Formula 14 and your journey to health a success, you must identify your emotional patterns, determine which ones are hurting your health, and align them to make you unstoppable on this journey. Take it from me, the former king of emotional eating and using food for all the wrong reasons, this is important. When people get this part right, they lose the weight in spite of themselves. They start a new diet or exercise regimen and stick to it because their emotions, which are more powerful than any logical reasons for becoming lean, support them instead of hindering them. The massive amounts of energy once used to obsess about food and continue the patterns that lead to being overweight are released and become a support system.

Do you have patterns that you use to add a little drama to your boring daily routine? When you are sitting in traffic on the way to work, do you get furious at the other drivers for the first half-hour, then pull into a fast-food restaurant, grab a sausage biscuit, hashbrowns, and coffee, and feel the calming effect as the food causes you to relax and your emotions are now centered and peaceful? Then, when you pull into the office, do you regret the breakfast you had? Do you eat healthy from Monday to Friday and then cut loose on the weekends? Are you a "foodie" whose main social identity is going to new restaurants and overeating regardless of the impact it has on your body? The thrill and delight when that fresh, new, visually stunning plate is laid before you are building neural pathways and habits that are hard to overcome. Starting a new diet or healthy lifestyle without a plan to redirect the emotional joy you get from being a "foodie" can cause a relapse in a few months, weeks, days, or even hours.

So many people live their daily lives filled with stress and the feeling of being overwhelmed. If food alleviates that stress three to six times a day, an emotional pattern is established that is burned into your nervous system, keeping you overweight.... it impacts your entire life. You don't have the energy and focus for your loved ones and the things that are really important. When your emotion is aligned with your goals and this journey creates passion in your life, you will not slide backward as often or for as long a period of time. Begin to capture your emotion and be its master instead of its victim.

Getting control of your mind and emotions is 80% of your weight loss journey. If a severely obese couple in their fifties received a video email of their daughter, who was being held captive, with demands that they both lose 100 pounds in the next six months or their daughter would die, all of their emotional power, their incredible love for their daughter, would eliminate any obstacle. They would run to their computer and quickly find people who had lost 100 pounds rapidly. Within five minutes, they would be on an intense diet and fitness plan. They would start losing weight within minutes, and they would both seemingly easily lose the 100 pounds. In other words, the compelling reason to act would enable them to be decisive about TAKING IMMEDIATE ACTION, wasting no time in getting the ball rolling towards saving their daughter. Contrast that with an email from their daughter telling them that she had seen a news report on type II diabetes and that she was worried about them and their eating habits. Many parents would respond, "Aww, that is so sweet. Pass me another cupcake, would you, honey?"

So first, let us examine what possible benefits you get from being overweight. Is it simply the freedom to eat whenever and whatever you want? Is there something deeper? Are you a polarity responder who got so sick of being lectured on your weight that you thumbed your nose up and got really heavy? Just having a grasp of any positive elements of being overweight can help you begin to weaken its power over you.

The first question you have to ask yourself is: What do I gain from being overweight?

If the answer isn't obvious at first, come up with as many possibilities as you can to find the hidden benefit that you get from being overweight. Is the "issue" a part of your identity? Does it make you feel loved when a family member says, "we are so worried about your weight." Is your weight a passive/aggressive instrument you benefit from? Once you find the answer, you must strip it of its power and replace the benefit with something healthy. For instance, if your weight makes you feel loved, then question that belief. Ask yourself, "What if I start having medical challenges or can't do some things because of my weight? Will that love turn to hate?" Does your weight give you an outlet for blame? Lack of money, lack of confidence: "It's the weight's fault, not mine."

There are six human needs identified by Chloe Madanes and Tony Robbins. They say if four or more of those needs are satisfied by something, you are compelled to do it. Overeating satisfies all of the six human needs for me:

I get CERTAINTY from food—planning what I am going to eat and when.

I get UNCERTAINTY from food—what will I change today and eat differently? Endless choices of food.

I get SIGNIFICANCE from food—look at me and my issue! This is so hard! What am I going to do about my weight? Let's discuss this. I get LOVE/WARMTH from food. Breaking bread for 53 years with friends and family. Wonderful meals at grandparents. With my family. Golden Buddha, The Club. Lullwater-Tavern. Crab Trap. Barbara Jean's. Waffle House. Red Lobster.

I get LEARNING AND GROWTH—new diets, new strategies, another issue to solve. More to discuss with friends and family.

I get CONTRIBUTION as I rush to get Subway, Mellow Mushroom, Zaxby's, Starbucks, Dunkin', chocolate, and snacks for family members. Even on a 40-day fast I am preparing food for family.

How can I fulfill these needs another way? I am CERTAIN the principles of Formula 14 will lead to a more fulfilling life. They will be my solid foundation, my certainty.

UNCERTAINTY: Learn to explore and cook new foods/recipes. Make the variety and spontaneity healthy choices instead of destructive ones.

Get SIGNIFICANCE by being a beacon of health and helping others get healthy too. Instead of moaning and groaning about "my terrible health," I can be positive and uplifting.

Get LOVE/WARMTH by communing over healthy foods or communing over physical activities and no food at all!

GROWTH from finding new ways to share Formula 14, and

CONTRIBUTION by doing nice things for people that, if they involve health, it's positive and not always unhealthy foods.

Next, let's dive deep and brainstorm to create a list of "whys" that you are committed to reaching your ideal weight. Come up with 14 powerful reasons that you will stay within your F14# and never damage your body by overeating again. Some examples:

MY FAMILY. My children: being overweight is setting a terrible example for them. To be there for my children and grandchildren for as long as possible. My wife: she has endured through the years. She stood by me for the first 22 years; make the next 40 fun, romantic, and incredible.

ILLNESS. HEART DISEASE: a friend's heartbreaking heart attack experience recently. Being on the phone with them and hearing their cries of anguish as they lost their dad/husband. They were in the ambulance on the phone all the way through to the doctor, informing them of his death. Keith's heart attack. CANCER: Laura was ravaged by the time she was diagnosed. Hamilton. Ad. Dandy. Mema. Dana. David. Mom's struggle with two hard battles. DIABETES: my eyes, my kidneys. My neighbor who is dealing with MS through no fault of her own, while I used to take actions—self-inflicting damage that could cause fatal or catastrophic health events at a young age.

GOD. My body is a temple, a gift from God. I will honor that instead of desecrating it. I will realign with my faith and get on a spiritual path.

CONFIDENCE. I am much more confident when I am lean.

Being an ACTION MAN… a doer, not a talker. TO PRACTICE WHAT I TEACH. The momentum I will get by finally accomplishing something!

ENERGY AND VITALITY to fuel an amazing life. I will have the energy to be a great husband, dad, son, brother, and friend at the same time. I will have the energy to succeed at work, at play, and in my relationships.

MONEY. The first 53 years of my life have been focused on food. Create new momentum, and instead of focusing on the next meal take care of my family with more financial stability.

PHYSICAL FITNESS. To finally be able to thrive and accomplish physical fitness goals, and have an active lifestyle.

To be a positive example and help friends and family be healthier instead of a warning as obesity destroys my life. Mark Twain says the two most important days in your life are the day you were born and the day you figure out why.

Have the resources to travel and have fun again.

THE NAYSAYERS. All the people who giggle and think to themselves, "He is going to gain all of his weight back. He will always be fat." PROVE THEM WRONG!

Brainstorm now, come up with your reasons, and return to this section.

Now, go through your list of compelling reasons why you are committed to reaching your ideal weight, and pick one that is your overarching reason. This is what you draw on when you feel like returning to your old patterns or breaking your F14#. (And remember, if you do, simply forgive yourself IMMEDIATELY and jump back on and recommit the next meal or the next day).

There is a saying I've heard, "If your why doesn't make you cry, then it's not strong enough." Whatever works for you, whatever helps you stick with your weight loss, use it. There is no one way. One person may go to a high school reunion and overhear an old classmate whisper, "Jane has gained so much weight!" The next day, Jane sets off on a furious mission and loses 50 pounds in two months. Another person may get a bad report from their doctor. We've all heard the stories of the children who said to their daddy, "Please stop smoking; I want you to be alive when I graduate from college," and the man quits that day. Find your "why." It isn't easy. Behaviors that have been ingrained since childhood can be hard to break. Formula 14 made it easier for me, because having the maximum calorie limit allowed me to be more lenient in some areas of consumption, giving me a wide variety of choices within that limit.

Let me tell you another secret. Your "why" does not have to be real. Remember the Michael Douglas movie called *The Game* , where he is pushed to the edge, and ultimately, his life is transformed by thinking he had lost everything? What if your doctor ran a bunch of tests and came back and told you, "You have severe heart disease and will be dead in six months if you don't make serious changes in your diet and begin to exercise." You are terrified and go on a major health kick. Two months later, your doctor tells you that your numbers are improving. You feel better and eventually get a clean bill of health.

Fifty years later, you are cleaning out your attic and find a letter addressed to your wife. The letter is from the doctor who scared you straight all those years ago. "I hope your husband is doing well," the letter says, "I felt bad about tricking your husband and making him think that he was in danger of dying, but I understand he is over 90 years old now." You discover that your labs were not terrible, but they had shifted a little and that your doctor told you that you had serious health problems because your wife begged him to. She was concerned about your poor eating habits and sedentary lifestyle, so she made a deal with your doctor. You realize that your "why" was never real.

Perhaps this is a silly example in today's sue-happy culture, but would you be grateful you were still alive because of the lifestyle changes you made, or would you feel cheated that you could have continued to destroy your health and died 30 years ago? You would probably smile and be happy that your wife cared enough about you to scare you straight. The point I am making here is that the only person who has to believe in your "why" is you. Find the reasons you need to propel you forward and turn them into convictions.

People are always looking for the magic pill or gimmick that will make them leaner and healthier. I have finally discovered the secret, and I'm now ready to reveal it to you on this very page. I have a secret strategy that will make you lean and give you an abundance of energy. Are you ready? It's you. You are the secret ingredient. Everything you need to accomplish this goal is already inside of you right now, at this very moment. Take action and make Formula 14 work for you!

CHAPTER 11
FORMULA 14 PHASE 11
(HOUR 11/DAY 11/WEEK 11)

IDENTITY SHIFT PART TWO: THE TWO PATHS MEDITATION, REPLACEMENT BEHAVIORS.

I could have been someone!
Well so could anyone
You took my dreams from me
When I first found you

I kept them with me, babe
I put them with my own
Can't make it all alone
I've built my dreams around you

The boys of the NYPD choir
Still singing "Galway Bay"
And the bells are ringing out
For Christmas Day

Fairytale of New York - The Pogues

TWO PATHS MEDITATION

Let's continue to work on mindset and shifting identity. To begin the two paths meditation set your phone timer for 7 minutes, sitting quietly with your eyes closed, and picturing the next 14 years if you do nothing to change your health. Be candid and brutal with yourself about what could happen if you continue to remain overweight. For example, when I did this, I pictured falling down dead while playing with my son. He shook me, but I was gone, and the trauma destroyed his life over the next twenty years until it ended badly, too. I did this with other serious health conditions, which really jolted me.

Now, set the timer for 7 minutes, close your eyes, and picture the opposite. Imagine you embrace your F14# and follow it rigidly. There are some slip-ups along the way, but you eventually shed the weight, engage in physical activities you love, and attract the partner of your dreams if you are single, your health spirals upward, and in 14 years, you are living an incredible life! Draw on these images when times are tough, and remember the two paths and where you want to go.

REPLACEMENT BEHAVIORS

Replacement behaviors are important because if your life revolves around food, overeating, and bingeing on Netflix, you will need to fill the void. Back when tons of people smoked, you may remember most people who quit smoking gained an enormous amount of weight. Many of them replaced cigarettes with snacking on potato chips and Candy. With Formula 14, you have a large selection of replacement behaviors in the upcoming phases. Aerobic exercises, free hand exercises, and different eating strategies to replace the old ones. If you are a meat lover, split the large steak with your spouse or a friend and have a double order of broccoli with it instead of a buttery potato and the bread they bring out before your meal.

If you get stressed at work, sit in your car at lunch and do a Flight, Fight, or Thrive session and/or some deep breathing for 14 minutes before you rush to a fast food restaurant for some comfort food.

Make this a fun process and simply start filling the old schedule with new and empowering activities.

If you think, "I'm going to go over my calories and have a large steak with Parmesan butter crust and fries instead of a sweet potato," initiate a replacement behavior if possible. You will make a list of 14 replacement behaviors in phase 14.

Make a list of replacement behaviors that could work for you. You may want to complete this list once you have explored the other phases of Formula 14.

Many of mine are from later phases of Formula 14, so you will have a better understanding once you have read those sections. Here is my list of Replacement Behaviors:

1. Power Phrases: Shout, speak, write, read, or listen to a power phrase.
2. Leisurely hike or walk with family, friends, or dogs, or a structured cardio session.
3. Deep breathing or alternate nostril breathing
4. Mini or Full FFT session.
5. A healthier food than the one I wanted, or a much smaller portion than usual.

6. Drink some water instead of eating.
7. A mini fast. Instead of eating ________, I will skip and intermittently fast until _____am/pm.
8. Resistance exercises. If one of the body parts is being worked that day, do that free-hand exercise instead of eating.
9. Work activity that would help take care of my family and get my mind off of eating.
10. Spend time with my wife or do
11. Something nice for her. Do a spontaneous activity or date, or engage in intimacy, or work on the house, yard, or car.
12. Spend time with the kids.
13. Call or spend time with a friend or family member.
14. Crank some music and envision any of your power phrases being completed/achieved. Sing!
15. Close your eyes and think about the overarching reason why you are losing weight!

CHAPTER 12
FORMULA 14 PHASE 12

(HOUR 12/DAY 12/WEEK 12)

LAYERING STRATEGIES (EXTERNAL FORCES, THE EXTREMES, MAGNIFICENT EVENTS, LORDS OF DISCIPLINE, THE TORTOISE AND THE HARE)

Oh, you never learned the 'Whens' and 'Wheres' and 'Whys'
And I still believe that you were dying to be everything
To everyone and for all time
Ah, the golden boy did you stop trying?
Did it turn out stale, or did it simply lose its wonder?
Could you hold it up from out and under?
Does the distance seem to dim-dumb-dim your memory?
Does the distance seem to fell the hunger?

Something to Say - The Connells

Creating unstoppable momentum requires aligning your emotions and your mind. Here are the strategies you can use to combine these forces. These strategies can give you a boost when it comes to your energy and emotional power, and tapping into your willpower. So, what are the effective emotional and mental motivators that can guide people to their weight loss goals? They are:

External Forces. My wife pressing me to "just admit you can't do anything and get gastric bypass" pushed me to take action. That is an example of an external force propelling me forward to accomplish my goal. Another external force would be a doctor saying, "Based on these tests, you will be dead in two years if you don't change your diet and start moving." This will give most people the pressure they need to make a shift. Heart disease, diabetes, and other serious health conditions can be powerful motivators to bring about change.

The Extremes. Diet and exercise plans that many would consider radical are what I call the Extremes. These are diet and exercise plans that are incredibly difficult and hard to stay on for long periods of time. Fasting, colon cleanses, extreme low carb/no carb, ultramarathons, etc. These diet and exercise plans are challenging to start, somewhat painful to stick with, and almost impossible to maintain forever. My extremes would be running a half marathon with very little training or a 21-day, 30-day, and 40-day water-only fast.

But when it comes to the difficulty of sticking with anything, time can wear you down, and your willpower can collapse. That is the reason the Atkins Diet begins adding back more carbohydrates after the induction period. Living on meat, eggs, and two cups of veggies each day is incredibly clogging and acidic, but as a short-term corrective measure, it can be incredibly beneficial to some people, especially if they were addicted to French fries and sugary drinks.

Magnificent Events. Weddings, high school reunions, weight loss contests, etc., can be powerful motivators. As you push yourself to run up each hill, you tell yourself, "I have been planning this wedding for two years. This is one of the biggest days of my life. I WILL LOOK GOOD FOR IT!" A word of warning about magnificent events: the day after. Many people who enter weight loss contests say to themselves, "When this is over, I am going to eat a large pizza and ten brownies!" So, the second you reach your goal, you are starting the destructive process to reverse it.

I knew a man who went to the Betty Ford Clinic for alcohol addiction, and he told me something very powerful and profound. He said that they did not tell you when you would be leaving. That way, you are not sitting around saying, "Just three more weeks, and I can have a drink." I remember when I awarded myself for achieving a weight loss goal at a magnificent event—with a double doozie (a huge glob of icing mashed between two cookies) from the Great American Cookie Company™! Don't let the event be the ending. Rather, make it the beginning. If you lose 50 pounds for your wedding, have a delicious dinner and a big piece of wedding cake, shake your groove thing on the dance floor (and in the hotel room) for a few hours, and then make sure you have a salad with every meal on your honeymoon. Take long walks on the beach and transition to the next strategy for losing or maintaining. And always remember your F14#!

Lords of Discipline Some people can use raw willpower and determination to achieve their goals. This willpower aligns their emotions, and they are off to the races! When my brother decides to lose weight, he can immediately start eating healthier and exercising. I remember having to hem and haw, have five last suppers, read new books, and contemplate what strategies I should use. If you have the willpower to make the shift, use it. After about three weeks, the raw willpower will give way to new habits. The results will be displayed on the scale, in the mirror, or even by a good report from your doctor.

An Ode to Willpower Years ago, I saw an episode of *Monster in Law* on the A&E Network. An obese man was being tormented by his mother-in-law to lose weight. "Don't put so much mayonnaise on that," she scolded him repeatedly, and "You are my TON-in-law." He was obese, and she was riding him hard to make a change. She had lost her husband and did not want her daughter to lose hers, too, so her intentions were good, but the situation was spiraling out of control, and someone was going to have to move out. The mother-in-law was blasting him because she couldn't understand why he didn't just use a little willpower and lose the weight. When I would discuss the latest diet or exercise plan, a comedian I knew used to say, "Eat a salad!" Is it really that easy? Maybe. Maybe not. What if self-control and willpower are inborn to some degree and then must be cultivated to be successful with it?

The now-famous marshmallow study by Walter Mischel seems to strongly support the importance of willpower and built-in self-control. Four-year-old children were given a marshmallow, and before the adult left the room, they were offered a deal—if they denied themselves the instant gratification of eating the marshmallow and didn't eat it for 15 minutes, they could have two marshmallows. You can guess what happened. Years later, the children who exercised their willpower and self-control were much more successful: better grades, better SAT scores, and higher salaries when they started their careers. [1]

What if it all really just came down to good old-fashioned willpower, and if you have it, you have it, and if you don't, you don't? I think that may be the launch pad, the beginning, but I believe willpower has a finite reserve and will eventually collapse if additional steps are not taken. Replacement behaviors literally wire your new habits and make them second nature. In the beginning, they will build enough willpower to get you through the first few crucial weeks of reprogramming. So what if the four-year-old children who denied the marshmallow were about to deny the keg parties at college and chose to study instead. It was hard for a few weeks, but eventually, it was easier. Formula 14 allows you to use your willpower to stick to the plan and to also have the freedom to eat whatever you want sometimes.

One of the best strategies to keep a person on track to attain their goals is to do a 30-Day Formula 14 Power Push. You can stick to almost anything for 30 days! You embedding a goal in a 30-day period to give yourself some momentum, which will ultimately create a habit. Then, your actions will be second nature, and you won't need willpower. With Formula 14 as a baseline, a rigid diet that one would normally consider extreme could be beneficial. What would you be willing to stick to for 30 days with good old-fashioned willpower? Your answer could change your life. Even if it's "nothing." Especially if it's "nothing!"

Willpower alone is not enough, but raw willpower can even-

---

1. Baumeister, Roy F. and John Tierney. Willpower: Rediscovering the Greatest Human Strength, The Penguin Press, 2011, pg. 10

tually lead to new habits forming. This long-term change can mean a total transformation.

A few words about structure, discipline, and rebelling against the rigid guidelines of most diets. The structure that plagued me and made me instinctively rebel had to be removed before I could successfully lose weight. Some people are wired differently and need rigid guidelines: a piece of toast and a hard-boiled egg for breakfast, a turkey sandwich on whole grain bread with one packet of low-fat mayonnaise for lunch, etc. I'm wired a little differently. I am a contrarian, or what Richard Bandler, the co-investor of Neuro Linguistic Programming, would call a polarity responder. He discovered this when he got a speeding ticket in England. He went to court and noticed that everyone was trying to argue their way out of their tickets and the judge was instantly taking the opposite stand and declaring them guilty. So when Bandler was called forward, he said (I am paraphrasing here), "Your honor, I was speeding, and I am guilty, guilty, guilty! I deserve the maximum penalty!" The judge paused and then said, "Well, wait a minute, Dr. Bandler, why were you in a hurry?"

So, since I know how I am wired, I can use that to my benefit and create pressure to propel me toward my weight loss goals. A rigid plan will work for me for a few days (or even hours). Then, I will cast it aside and embrace my newfound "freedom," which is really an excuse to eat whatever I want. So, the F14# is incredibly helpful to me: a target range that has a relaxed feeling of flexibility. Remember, when you set rigid guidelines, the restriction itself becomes the magnet for repeating the old behaviors. Take the opposite approach. Acknowledge that you can have french fries whenever you want to.... there are mountains of them everywhere, fast food joints beckoning from every other intersection, but since it has not been categorized as a "forbidden fruit," it loses its grip on the psyche. I spent almost twenty years obsessed with last suppers. "I am about to be really rigid and strict, so I am going to eat a giant platter of fried seafood and a loaded baked potato tonight, then have a delicious treat before bedtime. The next day, the rigid diet feels horrible, and since I have mastered diet and exercise strategies and know everything I need to do (with rigid discipline and precision), it is okay to break down and eat whatever I want. But TOMORROW is really, really, really, really, really going to be the day! I am going to go all out, so I guess I better plan another last supper for tonight." I am embarrassed to admit that I lived in that pattern for years, and my weight ballooned up to 361 pounds.

The exciting thing for anyone who has struggled with their weight for years is that they have an amazing adventure ahead of them—if they frame it that way. If torture and misery are what you perceive, then torture and misery are what you will achieve. You have the ability to find out what makes you tick, identify the habitual patterns that have added excess weight to your frame, and begin to make the mental shifts in your life that will impact your health forever. I am not saying it will be easy—it could be the hardest thing you have ever done. Neural pathways have been created in your brain: superhighways geared toward keeping you fat. Let's annihilate them with Formula 14 and create superhighways to new health and energy!

The opposite ends of the spectrum are often the same. You can be blinded by complete darkness or an abundance of light. Achieving a healthy existence can be accomplished the same way: the Olympian with a rigid training schedule at one extreme and Forrest Gump running aimlessly from coast to coast at the opposite end of the spectrum. Both have an amazing level of fitness. I needed to realize that there truly is freedom in discipline, and it does not contradict spontaneity.

Spontaneously lying around all day and using pizza, ice cream, and brownies to create some flexibility in the tummy is not a good thing!

NO LAUGHING MATTER

I was a fan of *The Biggest Loser*™ TV show on NBC. If you are not familiar with the show, a group of obese individuals compete to lose as much weight as possible and win $250,000.00. They go through intense training sessions and restrict their calories. The workout sessions and weigh-in segments of the show are fun to watch, but the dialogue and psychological issues are the most interesting and helpful to me. In season 12 of the show, an obese man named Vinny was joking around with members of his team, pretending that his giant belly could talk. He named his bombastic belly "Cecil" and was mashing the fat around his belly button to make it appear like Cecil could talk. The team trainer was introduced to Cecil and was not amused. He said that the fat was going to kill Vinny and that he should be serious about getting healthy.

This scene made me realize that I had the same problem. I was always joking around at work, walking past people's offices with the front of my shirt pulled over my head to expose my enormous belly. They would find this hilarious and start laughing, but now I realize that the joke was on me and my health. I was using humor to hide the seriousness of my physical situation, and it was no laughing matter. This does not mean that you can't be light, cheerful, and even goofy sometimes. I was not fun to be around every time I started a new diet and exercise program. I was serious and miserable. I was beginning to detox, craving the foods that had made me fat. People around me could tell by the look on my face that I was not in the best state of mind. So, I am not saying you must be stoic, serious, and miserable as you begin to shift your thinking and your lifestyle. But do you joke around and attempt to divert the focus from your physical situation? Take some time to explore this, and you may be surprised.

In many ways, the war I have waged against emotional eating, carb addiction, laziness, and diet madness has been a self-absorbed and all-consuming, and that may be the problem. Deepak Chopra tells a story about a man who went to study enlightenment at a monastery in the Far East. When the new student asks the master how long it will take to learn the lessons of enlightenment, the master says, "Seven years." The student is upset by this projection and tells the master, "You don't understand. I will do whatever it takes to master this stuff. I will work all day and night and be completely consumed to make this happen. I will force myself to do whatever it takes." The master is quiet for a moment, weighing the words of his new student, and says, "Fourteen years then." The struggle, the battle, the obsession with being consumed with diet, exercise, and health can block a person from taking action—paralysis by analysis.

The Tortoise and the Hare (Baby Steps vs. Giant Leaps): The tortoise is slow and deliberate but can be the perfect strategy for those who resist dramatic change. Ultimately, the tortoise can be healthier in the long run. If I had started making tiny changes a decade ago and only lost a pound every two months, I would have been 100 pounds lighter. One of my personal trainers always said, "The fastest way to lose weight is slowly."

During my 40-plus years fighting the battle of the bulge, I have yo-yoed back and forth between embracing dramatic change or incremental change. There are very convincing arguments for both approaches, and a little introspection is required to figure out what combination works best for you. The best option is an innovative, dramatic change combined with small steps that create building blocks for long-term success. Each phase of Formula 14 has builds on each other. You could read through the book and start them all at once with total immersion, do a phase each day over 14 days, or take it slow and implement a phase each week.

Incremental Change (Baby Steps): Incremental change can be effective because it allows you to trick your fight-or-flight impulse and ease into a new and healthy lifestyle. Instead of saying, "This is it. Tomorrow I am going to start running, lifting weights, and eating a raw food diet," waking up, feeling overwhelmed, and doing nothing, you can take smaller steps, build momentum, and create great results in your health and fitness. Some examples: What if you ran to the first telephone pole on your street? The next day, you ran to the second telephone pole. The third day, you ran to the third telephone pole and only ate one scoop of ice cream before bed instead of two. The fourth day, you did five pushups against the wall after your run. The fifth day, you replaced the morning donut with a bagel with sugar-free jelly. Within a month, these incremental changes have created unstoppable momentum as new habits have been formed. In the book "One Small Step Can Change Your Life," author Dr. Robert Maurer recalls a patient he was working with who was overweight and stressed. A fellow doctor recommended that she (the patient) begin to exercise. Maurer realized that she was overwhelmed and suggested, "How about if you just march in place in front of the TV set for one minute each night?" The doctor gave him a disapproving stare, but the lady brightened. She agreed to do it. The time she spent walking in place increased. At her next office visit, she asked, "What else can I do for a minute?" Within a few months, her negative associations with exercise had been replaced with a love for movement, and she started aerobics classes. [2]

Dramatic Change (Giant Leaps): The best argument for dramatic change is that you can get rapid results, which tells you, "This is working!" With the slow, steady, and often unrewarding march of incremental change, you won't see any major results for quite some time. When I lost 87 pounds in 16 weeks during a weight loss contest, I was rewarded every Saturday at the weigh-in. I was getting the support of my friends and family because I would text the results to everybody after each weigh-in. This enabled me to stay focused.

Dramatic change can be fleeting and temporary, so it is important to remember the overarching "why" that motivates you. I used to be convinced that the best option for me was dramatic change. At one point, I decided to attempt gradual changes. I was convinced that I could slowly increase my water intake, slowly switch to healthier foods, and begin an exercise program. At the same time, I would slowly decrease my high glycemic carbs, portion amounts, etc. At the end of the first month, I had only lost 9.75 pounds. That is mot real rewarding when you are morbidly obese. I decided to document every ounce of water, every calorie, and every gram of carb/protein, and make sure that each day I was increasing the good and decreasing the bad. This was a lesson in futility. Going from large fries to medium and back to large was accomplishing nothing. A smaller amount of French toast still left me craving sweet breakfast food. Shifting from a Grande (medium) Strawberries and Crème Frappuccino at Starbucks™ to a Tall (small), then to

---

2. Maurer, Robert, PhD. One Small Step Can Change Your Life, Workman, 2006, pg. 16

a Tall with a slice of Banana Walnut Bread accomplished nothing.

Even though rapid change is dramatic and rewarding, it can boomerang, especially if you are using discomfort, fear, or anger to move you forward. When my weight loss contest was over, and the possible embarrassment of a poor showing was removed, I slowly started to regain weight. Sweet tea, coffee drinks, and shakes would replace much of my water consumption. When my weight gain hit the 15 to 20-pound mark, I would shift from sugary drinks back to water and move back down to the weight I was at the end of the contest. Then, I would get comfortable again and abandon the healthier lifestyle, and start to gain again. Why did this happen? There was no joy and fulfillment, nothing I was moving towards that was building new behaviors and habits. There was no longer a goal to achieve. For example, several times, I have been terrified by a physical ailment that has motivated me to take action. A pain in my shin that I believed was a stress fracture, and if I didn't get some pounds off, it would never heal. Dizziness. Is my pancreas shutting down? Nodding off in the middle of the day. Numbness in the morning. Diabetes? Fear stirs me to action, and I quickly drop 30 pounds. When the symptoms go away, the motivation to stay the course is removed. This is the pattern that so many people experience. I feel terrible with this excess weight; I am going on a diet and will start walking. Three weeks later: "I feel so much better. I am going to celebrate tonight with some pizza and beer." The next morning: "I feel terrible. Let's go get some breakfast. Pancakes, eggs, sausage, and coffee would be delicious and will pick me up a little." That afternoon, exercise is skipped and the weight gain cycle has returned. You know yourself better than anyone. You know what will work best for you: dramatic change, baby steps, or a combination. This will build momentum for you and lead you to your ideal weight. To eventually feel great about yourself, Formula 14 will begin to address the underlying issues causing emotional eating. You will begin to make the right choices, which will lead you to take the right actions. A combination of dramatic change and baby steps would mean taking massive action and working on turning the fundamentals into habits.

The way to get the process started is to notice your patterns and find ways to make implementing the Phases of Formula 14 fun. I love to crank music in my headphones when I am on the treadmill or elliptical. I imagine being at a concert instead of just staring at the wall and saying to myself, "This is so boring." Make the things you need to do pleasurable and fun, while making the things that hurt you harder and burdensome. Procrastinate on things that impede your progress. Love cookies? Procrastinate on making them. Say, "Maybe tomorrow," and make sure you don't have the ingredients at home to make them!

Before Formula 14, incremental change always led me back to overeating and a sedentary lifestyle. It stems from emotional eating and carb addiction. After one lengthy period of weight loss, I decided to start eating bran muffins. Bran muffins became bran muffins with butter. Bran muffins with butter became blueberry muffins. Blueberry muffins became cookies... and on and on. I was determined to use incremental change to improve my health. I experienced a little weight loss and then, a month later, was back at my starting weight. Not real impressive! By having the calorie ceiling as the overarching principle in Formula 14, I can't backslide like that. Even if I have a bad night calorie-wise out to dinner with friends, I can be right back on the path the next morning.

Dramatic change on a whim has only happened once, and

that was when I decided to become a vegetarian. A friend of mine was a vegetarian and made a good case, so I just stopped eating meat one day. I didn't say, "Next Monday is the day I am swearing off meat forever!" I just did it. That was a unique experience for me, though. I am a dramatic change kind of guy, but I need an overwhelming why. I build it up. The main reason is because I usually need an external force to propel me forward. Anthony Robbins, the successful author and life coach, talks about how some people use internal representations and others use external representations. I am motivated by the external. When my employer offered to pay for my training and gym membership if I wanted to be in the biggest loser contest, there was no way I would let them down and not use it and not compete with intensity. Having an external representation can be helpful, but it can also backfire once the external force has been removed. People who are internally motivated can "do it for their own reasons and by their own personal compass." One way Robbins suggests that you determine what representation system you use is to ask yourself, "How do I know that I did a good job?" Do you just know internally, or do you need a boss or co-worker to tell you, "You did a really good job!" When making a decision, do external opinions exercise a major influence on you, or do you reach your own conclusions and know what path you want to take? Do you predominantly use internal or external representations? How could you leverage your representations to keep you focused on your objectives? And finally, how can you leverage internal and external representations, and positive and negative reinforcement to accomplish your goals?

ALL OR NOTHING THINKING One thing to watch for with dramatic change is it can fall into the category of all or nothing thinking and severely damage your progress. Here's why: Two weeks after embarking on a serious weight loss journey, you break down at a birthday party and have some cake. "I ruined my diet," you think to yourself after finishing the plate. The next morning, you skip the grapefruit and choose instead to have the Sunday brunch buffet. This leads to a Thanksgiving-style 90-minute session of eating omelets, waffles, chocolate-dipped strawberries, biscuits, bacon, sausage, and plenty of coffee to keep you awake once the binge session has ended. This leads to more guilt, and you think to yourself, "Since I am going to go back on my diet tomorrow, I'm going to have pizza tonight because I missed it." All of this started with a piece of birthday cake! A friend told me that her nutritionist said to her, "If you get a flat tire, do you jump out of the car and flatten the other three?" No. You fix the flat and continue down the road. The morning after the birthday cake, you could have had the brunch and eaten fresh fruit and a vegetable omelet, or even pancakes, but stayed within your calories, and your weight loss and journey back to health would have continued.

Steve Prefontaine was an elite runner from Oregon who almost won Gold in the 1972 Munich Olympics. ALMOST is the key word here, because he attempted to leave everybody in the dust (a human Secretariat), but he burned out late in the event. He was winning the race until the last 150 meters. Three runners passed him, and he was denied even earning the bronze a mere ten meters from the finish. Dr. David Burns, the famous psychologist who wrote the book *Feeling Good,* said that when you make it all or nothing, you often end up with just that... nothing. Look within and decide how you want to approach Formula 14. Consider each Phase, decide what will work best for you individually, and be flexible in your approach.

CHAPTER 13
FORMULA 14 PHASE 13
(HOUR 13/DAY 13/WEEK 13)

POWER PHRASING

Daylight turns to moonlight
And I'm at my best
Praising the way it all works
Gazing upon the rest
The cool before the warm
The calm after the storm
The cool before the warm
The calm before the storm

I wish to stay forever
Letting this be my food
But I'm caught up in a whirlwind and
My ever changing moods

The Style Council - My Ever Changing Moods

FORMULA 14 POWER PHRASING VISUALIZED AND INTERNALIZED

A power phrase is basically a passionate incantation that states a goal you want to achieve in the present tense. This will seem silly to most people, and I judged it harshly myself over the decades, even though it was recommended several different times by people I respected immensely. I don't know why this works. I don't know if it tunes your reticular activating system into things you need to do, if it's your action flows from the focus you are putting on these things, or if you simply can't be wondering about what fast food you are going to have for lunch if you are filling your mind with these phrases. I only ask that you act on this with an open mind and see if it works for you like it did for me.

Use your ideal weight to create your main Power Phrase:

"I weigh ______ pounds, and I feel incredible!!!"

Now create 3 additional Power Phrases that pertain to your health(energy, physical fitness, general health)

Then create 10 power phrases for other areas of life that need improvement. Mine were mainly financial, but they could address relationships, emotional control, things you are learning, etc.... (I am fluent in Chinese, and it has doubled my income!) these could be other areas you could explore.

Start with the main Power Phrase and record yourself saying it over and over on your phone. Use emotion and enthusiasm when you record the power phrase. Ultimately you want that audio file to include 100 impressions (you saying the power phrase 100 times with emotion). This is for convenience because we will be going through each power phrase in increments of 100 and then moving to the next, etc. At first, though, when you name the file, put the number of times you said it at the end of the file name to make it easier to count each audio impression. In addition to listening to it, you will say it to yourself internally, read it, speak it, occasionally shout it, and write it (use a journal or a notebook to record the written impressions). It's important to hear in the background, almost subliminally, but it's also important to consciously visualize the power phrase as being real. When you say your main power phrase, visualize yourself at your ideal weight and as having an abundance of energy surging through your body-the expression of feeling incredible.

As David R. Hawkins, M.D., Ph. D., says in his book, Healing and Recovery:

Picture the kind of body you want to have and the feeling you want to have about having this kind of body. Then, remember sometime in your life when you were feeling joyful and pleased with yourself. Next, picture the body the way you want it to be and re-awaken that emotion of joy. For example, if you want to be slim, picture yourself as slim and begin to love that picture of yourself. Love that picture of the body and then let it go, knowing that you have set up a program. You have set up what is going to happen in the future because the mind begins to move in that direction automatically. Just love that picture of yourself. If you like, you can put the number of pounds under it and picture how you want to look, and say, "You know it's fantastic to be slim and active and feel good about the body. I love myself for that." Research studies confirm that imaging techniques are effective. [1]

---

1. Hawkins, David R. Healing and Recovery, pg. 353-354, Veritas Publishing,

The visualization you occasionally do as you hear the power phrases should be very specific. Carry pictures of what your ideal body would look like, make it the screensaver on your phone, or carry the image in your head. Visualization can convince your mind that your lean body is not only on the way, it is the order of the day. When I was a lean 160 lbs in my twenties, I remember telling one of my friends that I had to do something about my weight, "It's getting out of control." He gave me a puzzled look and said, "I don't know what you mean." I lifted my shirt and pinched myself on the side, grabbing about a ¼ inch of skin. My friend simply shook his head. I also went to a Diet Center in downtown Decatur, Georgia, and told the consultant there that I needed to lose weight. She weighed me, and based on my height, I was in the perfect range, but I still wasn't getting it. Anyone who is thin but convinced that they are fat is destined to eventually be heavier once again.

You will be building the power phrases up thousands of impressions.

Begin each power phrase with the Formula 14 Subliminal, physical, and emotional Flood. This Emotional Whirlwind will be two 14-minute continuous sessions (you will do this once a week afterward) of flooding your heart and mind with the power phrase. This will be two 14-minute whirlwinds of positivity and bliss. Get moving like you are at a private concert with your favorite artist. Shout your incantation, say it, feel it, get energized. Listen to your recording over and over, speak or shout along with it, and envision it as accomplished. You can have it going silently in the background while you envision it and say it to yourself over and over.

Sedona, Arizona, 2009)

Vary the impressions for each power phrase daily. Here is an example of how mine is listed in the notes on my cell phone:

"I weigh 190 pounds, and I feel incredible!"

Audio: 16,600
internal audio: 200
Spoken: 160
Shouted: 5
Written: 155
Read: 300

Total: 17,220

This will cement them into your subconscious and into your life.

Increase the impressions of each power phase until it's your reality, or no longer useful and needs to be modified. For example, you get to your ideal weight and realize you want more muscle mass. The original power phrase would need to be modified to the new ideal weight. Or you reach a financial goal of _______ dollars saved, so you need to increase it, etc.

Emotional Whirlwinds burn the power phrases into your psyche much faster. Do this by intense visualizations of the impressions when you can, and acting upon the power phrases you can do instantly—for example: you can't snap your fingers and have a six-pack, but if you are a business owner and say you are going to create 20 minutes of online promotional content per day that is a measurable objective you could implement immediately.

Once your first power phrases are either your reality or replaced with another goal, add other power phrases to transform your life.

After the initial immersion with two consecutive Emotional Whirlwinds, build to 14,000 impressions and then continue (140,000? 1.4 million?) until the power phrases are your reality.

CHAPTER 14
FORMULA 14 PHASE 14
(HOUR 14/DAY 14/WEEK 14)

IDENTITY SHIFT PART FOUR: ALIGNING YOUR WORDS AND ACTIONS, TAKING TOTAL RESPONSIBILITY, THE SELF INTEGRITY SNOWBALL

Get some honesty
Take the best of me and then the rest let go
In every situation, with its tireless rage
Step outside your cage and let the real fool show

I should have stayed round to break the ice
I thought about it once or twice
But nothing ever changes
Unless there's some pain...

Tears for Fears - Goodnight Song

ALIGNING YOUR WORDS AND ACTIONS, THE RESPONSIBILITY PLEDGE, THE SELF INTEGRITY SNOWBALL

"This is it," I told my sister, Lane. "I am taking control of my health once and for all. I am signing a pledge to you that I am going to lose 100 pounds." My sister was supportive, but she probably knew that my words were hollow. I had that same conversation dozens of times over the years with my friends, family, and co-workers. Every time I did this and then failed to take action, I not only lost credibility with others, but I also lost it with myself. Eventually, if our words are not aligned with our actions, they mean nothing.

Darren Hardy, the publisher of Success Magazine, makes the point perfectly in his book, *The Compound Effect*: "If there is a discrepancy between what you say and what you do, I'm going to believe what you do every time. If you tell me you want to be healthy, but you've got Doritos dust on your fingers, I'm believing the Doritos." [1]

We discussed incremental and dramatic change. If you are better suited for incremental change, make minor claims and back them up with tiny actions, then gain momentum as your words and actions align. This will lead you to new habits and tremendous momentum.

For example, let's say Norma has a bowl of ice cream with hot fudge every night before bed. One afternoon, she announces to her husband that she has decided to lose 30 pounds. That night, he is surprised to see that the ice cream does not have fudge on it, but he thinks to himself, "She will never lose weight

1. Hardy, Darren. The Compound Effect, Success Media, 2010, pg. 76

this way." But two days later, the ice cream has been replaced with frozen yogurt. Ten days after that, she brings in a bowl of fruit. Two weeks pass, and then the nighttime fruit snack is replaced with a tall, cool glass of water! Norma made these seemingly small changes while boldly claiming each day that she was going to lose 30 pounds in the next six months.

Early on, a co-worker may have said, "How come you are eating that cheeseburger? I thought you said you were losing weight?" Norma smiles, "I've started walking in the morning, and my late-night bowl of ice cream with hot fudge has been replaced with water! I said my goal was 30 pounds in six months, not six weeks." Several weeks later, the cheeseburger becomes a tuna salad sandwich, then tuna salad on fresh greens. Her morning walk has become a three-mile jog. Breakfast is two eggs, and steamed broccoli with olive oil drizzled over the top. Norma achieves her goal, and she knows (as do her friends and family) that her word is as good as gold.

Aligning your words with your actions will increase your self-respect, confidence, and discipline. This builds positive momentum. The inverse is true as well. When your words mean little or nothing, your self-respect, confidence, and discipline falter, and your momentum spirals downward into unhealthy habits and actions.

Start bolstering your word today. If you are always 15 minutes late, surprise your friends and be the first one to the restaurant. If you have told your wife that you want to start going to bed earlier, surprise her by taking Advil PM™ when you pull into the driveway and then fall asleep at the dinner table with your face collapsed into your bowl of her famous spaghetti. JUST KIDDING! Go to bed a few minutes earlier every week, and eventually, you will be asleep much earlier (Easy for you to say, Jordan! I know, I know... getting to bed early is really hard for me). Formula 14 is a wonderful place to start making your word mean something again.

Also, remember to distinguish between promises you make to yourself and goals. Winning the softball championship is a goal, because there are elements of that that are beyond your control. The umpire could make bad calls, your star pitcher could catch the flu, etc., but promises you make to yourself, I will spend two hours per week in the batting cages, be at every practice unless there is an emergency, etc., are things you can control.

TAKING TOTAL RESPONSIBILITY:

A MENTAL CONUNDRUM: YOU MAY NOT BE COMPLETELY AT FAULT, BUT YOU MUST ACCEPT TOTAL RESPONSIBILITY FOR YOUR CURRENT CONDITION AND THE JOURNEY AHEAD.

In order to make a change, you will need to hold yourself accountable and accept total responsibility for everything pertaining to your health. This is difficult, especially with all the new research that tells us sometimes you may not be at fault! Dr. James McClernon of Duke University studies the brains of people who are addicted to drugs and has discovered that junk foods can stimulate the same response in the brain that powerful drugs can. So now you are screaming, "I had no idea that my soda and snack cakes were like crack and cigarettes, and you want me to accept total responsibility for my excess weight?"

Yes.

When you spread the blame around, a sense of helplessness can keep you stuck.

Which reaction to a bulging belly in the mirror is better? "I can't believe that society has set me up to be obese. I twisted my ankle and couldn't do my daily five-mile run, and now, six months later, I am fat. New studies show that some of these problems may start in the womb, with an obese mother, so it's not my fault!"

What if, without beating yourself up and making yourself fatter with a stress-induced surge of cortisol, you simply said, "I can't believe I let myself get fat. I should have lowered my calories drastically when I hurt my ankle and couldn't run anymore. I could have done a little exercise in the pool, too. Oh well, time to get busy and reverse course."

You have probably known someone who is a master of the blame game. Nothing is their fault. Their boss is taking advantage of them. Their lover doesn't understand them. Their wife is too demanding. Their mother-in-law is weakening their relationship. They never take responsibility for anything. I was a master of the blame game with my unsuccessful musical career. I was a singer in the 90s. My band toured the Southeast, and we thought we were wonderful. Legends in our own minds! We had a production deal at one of the major studios in Atlanta and almost sold out a 1,000-seat hall. A Vice President at one of the major record labels loved our music and would come to our shows. The label was not signing our style of music at that time, so nothing ever panned out with that avenue toward success.

According to my distorted sense of reality and need to affix blame on anyone but myself, the current trends and music styles were to blame. It was the label's fault, the industry's fault, and the changing music scene in Atlanta's fault. A healthier reaction early on would have been, "Where is our style of music popular?" "Should we be playing in Europe or at least approaching labels there?" "What other US labels may be interested in our style of music at this time?" Maybe we should have played music as a hobby and focused on building a traditional business where the odds of success were dramatically higher? Maybe I just didn't cut it as a singer! When the blame was affixed to anyone or anything other than me, I was stuck and had no chance of changing it.

When you accept total responsibility, you are telling yourself that you have the power to change things. You have the power to solve the problem. Even if your excess weight was a thyroid problem, would it be better to tell yourself that you had an awful disease and things were helpless and accept that you were going to be heavy, or would it be better to tell yourself that years of poor diet and exercise choices have now manifested themselves in a malfunctioning thyroid? Even if your belief wasn't accurate, would it be better to take total responsibility and start taking better care of yourself, or to say, "My thyroid is giving me problems, pass the meatloaf for a third serving, please!"

Playing the blame game will be impossible if you align your words and your actions. Each and every day, whenever you attempt to use excuses or the blame game, say loudly and proudly: I AM RESPONSIBLE!!! Yell it, scream it, shout it, dream it!!!

THE SELF INTEGRITY SNOWBALL (THE DF FRAMEWORKS FIRST COUSIN)

Now that you have absorbed the Formula 14 Program in its entirety, it's time to make some promises to yourself and keep them. Go back through each phase of Formula 14 and make a list of 7 "must do" actions, and a list of 7 of your "might do" actions. Mine were:

MUST DO

1. Consume less calories than my F14# each day, unless it's a strategically planned slightly heavier day to kick start my metabolism.
2. Follow the DF Framework and never break my F14# on a whim or unconsciously.
3. A minimum of 5 aerobic sessions per week and target at least one muscle group with the Home Tone Program.
4. Drink at least 70oz of water daily.
5. Do 14 Deep Breathing Exercises daily. Do 14 Alternate Nostril Breaths daily. Do 14 Calming Breaths Daily
6. Do 42 minutes of FFT Daily
7. Do 100 impressions of each of my Power Phrases Daily

MIGHT DO

1. Specific eating strategies within my daily allotted calories like DUODONICS, the feeding window, or a reset.
2. Stretch daily
3. 7000 to 14,000 steps daily
4. Increase my aerobic sessions from walking to jogging and running.
5. Complete the Appalachian Trail or a marathon
6. An extended water fast
7. Wake up at 5:00am after using the tortoise to slowly shift my sleep times.

The Self integrity Snowball will build momentum and reverberate throughout your entire life. The quality of being honest with oneself and acting in total alignment by staying consistent with your actions even when faced with challenges or the daily pressures of life. A person that has self-integrity upholds a standard by choosing to do what they say they will. This involves being authentic, accountable, and trustworthy to oneself and can have a greater impact on your life than any other phase of the Formula 14 Program. If you slip up, remember the DF Framework and forgive yourself, but never use that as a crutch not to build incredible momentum with The Self Integrity Snowball.

SECTION FOUR

THE PATH AHEAD

CHAPTER 15
A RECAP OF THE 14 PHASES

Don't tell me you don't know the difference
Between a lover and a fighter
With my pen and my electric typewriter
Even in a perfect world where everyone was equal
I'd still own the film rights and be working on the sequel.
And I'm giving you a longing look
Everyday
Everyday
Everyday I write the book

Every day I write the book - Elvis Costello

I COMPILED THE LIST OF THE 14 PHASES AND PLACED them in the notes on my phone. Having all the Phases in one place so I could make sure I was on track was incredibly helpful, so I included it below.

I also began to use what I call the F14 Audit: set two times throughout the day, mine are 11am and 6pm. In the calendar, you can set an alert at the time and five minutes before, so I made it 11:05am and 6:05pm, so I could have a reminder go off at the scheduled time and five minutes later so it couldn't be ignored.

Here is a recap of the 14 Phases of Formula 14:

THE CORE FOUR:

1. Formula 14 Master Principle: Your personal F14#. Ideal Weight X 14 = F14#.

2. Formula 14 Forgiveness Framework: Begin living your life within the F14# and later the other phases of Formula 14 by drawing a line in the sand with total DISCIPLINE. When you want to break down, think of your overarching "why" and see if this overrides the desire to break down. If you still want to break down, use one of your REPLACEMENT BEHAVIORS to replace the negative behavior. If this doesn't work and you still break down, forgive yourself IMMEDIATELY and get back on your F14# and the other phases.

3. Formula 14 Design Your Nutrition: Choose one (or a combination) of these:

- The Formula 14 Day Reset: Protein Masters.

- The Formula 14 Day Reset: Starch Masters.
- The Muscle Tone Formula.
- Formula 14 Fasting. Intermittent or Water Only
- DuoDonics For Life with a foundation of water-rich foods.
- The Diet of Your Choice.

4. Formula 14 Design Your Exercise: Work up to a minimum of 5 weekly sessions of 40 minutes in your aerobic zone and/or 7,000 to 14,000 steps 5 days per week. Find opportunities to move more. Choose a resistance system to build and retain muscle. Formula 14 Home Tone exercises, etc. Stretching routine.

THE FABULOUS FIVE:

5. Formula 14 Hydration. A minimum of five 14 oz servings of water daily.

6. Design your Supplementation. Determine what supplements, if any, work best for your body and consider using ClearDrops for systemic detoxification, Phix to fix your fat for good.

7. Breathing Exercises: A minimum of 14 deep breaths in the 1-4-2 ratio daily, 14 Alternate Nostril Breaths, and 14 Calming Breaths, daily!

8. Formula 14 Deep Sleep and Rest, Get on a consistent sleep schedule and make sure you are giving your body the rest it needs.

9. Stress Busting. FFT Sessions Build to three 14-minute sessions or 42 total minutes daily

THE FINAL FIVE: TRANSFORMATION WITH YOUR IDENTITY SHIFT

10. Identity Shift Part One (what I gain from being overweight, 14 reasons why, the overarching reason

11. Identity Shift Part Two: 14 Replacement Behaviors, The Two Paths Meditation

12. Identity Shift Part Three: Your Magnificent Event, External Forces, The Lords of Discipline, The Extremes, The Tortoise and the Hare

13. Identity Shift Part Four: Power Phrasing

14. Identity Shift Part Five: Aligning your Words and Actions, Taking Total Responsibility, The Self Integrity Snowball.

CHAPTER 16
WHAT ARE YOU GONNA DO?

Close the door, hold the phones, show me how…
Nothings ever gonna stop us now!

Cause we are, we are shining stars
We are invincible, we are who we are
On our darkest day, when we're miles away
So we'll come, we will find our way home

If you're lost and alone or you're sinking like a stone
Carry on
May your past be the sound of your feet upon the ground, and Carry on

Carry On - Fun

The time has come for you to make the decision to shift your identity and take control of your health. Let the old you fall by the wayside and become the healthy person that you envision and live your new lifestyle each and every day. And if the old you visits, the Forgiveness Framework shows them the door and quickly gets back to the new you.

When all is said and done, you will need self-discipline to begin the journey. Success coach Brian Tracy says that out of all the hundreds of success principles, the most important is self-discipline: doing what you know you should, even when you don't feel like doing it. Any goal you have comes down to the ability to follow through. Your core motivation is the catapult, but you release it and take the first step with self-discipline. [1] Take this journey with me. Decide today that you can and will reach your ideal weight with Formula 14.

The strategies in this book are just that: strategies. You are the missing ingredient. What is your "why"? What makes you tick? What will it take for you to realize that now is the time? Test Formula 14 on yourself. As for the other strategies in this book, think about them with an open mind and embrace the ones you find useful. For example, do not let people who have never dealt with being overweight destroy your ability to be as healthy as you can be. Remember this as you embark on a journey to get your health back. You know the old sun revolving around the earth cliché. New information is first ridiculed, then persecuted, then accepted, then praised.

For example, there are serious evolutionary biologists who believe that our primitive ancestors may have hunted their food by running it to death. While Neanderthals relied on spears and

1. Tracy, Brian, No Excuses, Vanguard Press, 2010, pp 6-7

clubs, we relied on our feet. This sounds preposterous because we are much slower than many of the animals we hunted, but when you examine the physiological factors, it makes perfect sense. A deer could easily outpace humans in a sprint, but many animals will quickly become oxygen-deprived and eventually collapse. One scientist, Dr. Dan Lieberman, determined that a man could run an antelope to death by scaring it into a gallop in hot weather. If the human can stay close and keep the antelope in sight, after about 6 miles, it will go into hyperthermia and collapse. Most of the people I know, if their survival depended on it, could learn to run 6 miles on a summer day. [2]

Right now, though, our survival may depend on losing excess fat. During the time it took you to read the paragraph above, an American grabbed their chest and suffered a heart attack. Three thousand Americans will suffer the same fate over the next twenty-four hours, about the same number of people who died in the 9/11 terrorist attacks. So take the step now and decide that you are going to determine what is best for your body. Get some compelling reasons and never look back. Make it happen for yourself and your loved ones.

2. McDougall, Christopher. Born to Run, Knopf, 2009, pp 227-228

www.ingramcontent.com/pod-product-compliance
Lightning Source LLC
LaVergne TN
LVHW041038150826
845672LV00001B/375

* 9 7 9 8 8 9 5 6 9 8 7 3 0 *